My Self, The Enemy

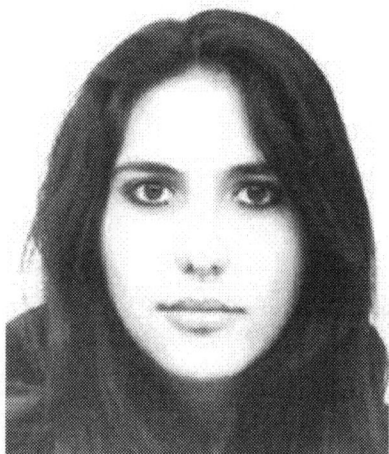

Published by:

Chipmunka publishing

PO Box 6872

Brentwood

Essex

CM13 1ZT

United Kingdom

www.chipmunkapublishing.com

Copyright © 2006 *Deborah Espect*

ISBN 978 1 84747 016 4

Foreword

"My Self, The Enemy" is written with startling honesty, openness and dry wit. The author writes with great candidness about depression, insecurity, work, relationships, social life, therapy and coming to terms with the diagnosis of Borderline Personality Disorder. 'My Self, The Enemy' is a raw novel written intelligently, sensitively and with a wry sense of humour.

About the Author:

Deborah Espect was born and raised in France and currently lives in East London. She has been through the mental health system in the UK and has drawn on her experiences to portray the huge emotional challenges that people with mental health issues have to face everyday. She was recently published in an American magazine and is currently working on a short film and a series of plays.

Acknowledgements

Many thanks to Mum, Monique, Yanik and Robyn for their love and support on this project.

Special thanks to Kathleen Bryson for all her helpful advice, Katherine Hayes and Joinedupwriters for making me believe in myself and coping with my mad ways.

Deborah Espect

Chapter 1

Why won't they leave me alone? There's always something. Always someone. The postman, the neighbours, the colleagues, don't they understand? I don't need anyone! Leave me in peace! Maybe I should move away. Find myself a nice house with a big, inaccessible field, or a forest, in the middle of nowhere. I'd grow my own vegetables, have a couple of cows to milk and I'd never need to see people ever again. What do they want from me anyway? It's not like I have anything to give. Because that's the thing, isn't it? No one asks how you are, what you're doing, if you had a nice weekend, out of kindness. They expect you to ask them the same. Attention seekers! But I'm not like them. I don't go around begging: 'Love me!' No wonder she has no friends, you probably think. Maybe I don't, but that's my choice. And I'm not completely alone, I have Naomi. We went to school together. Sometimes I think we only became friends because she didn't have anyone else to talk to either. Things haven't changed much since then. She used to be a complete nerd, and she still is. She's been at university for three years, doing a master or something; I never went. I was planning to be a vet, but the thought of killing anything, by duty or accident, terrified me. So did the idea of having to deal with the owners of the animals.

Sometimes I wish I had gone to university. Now I could do something more interesting than working in a crappy telephone survey company. But I couldn't handle more years of reading, researching and exams, not knowing whether there would even be a job at the end of it. I got this one out of luck, really. I saw an advert in the papers three years ago, just after I'd finished my A

Levels, when I was still living at my parents' in Kent. It said they were looking for people with 'No previous experience necessary', which came in handy since I'd never worked before; so I called them and all I had to do was go on a training course, and then I get the job! I'm quite good on the telephone; I don't have to see anyone I speak to, so I'm much more confident. Obviously, there are people around me in the office, but I don't talk to them. It's not the best wage in the world, but at least I'm doing something. Right? I don't know for how long I'll be in this job, but to be honest, I'm not sure what else I could do. I'm not good at much.

Naomi says I should try to set up my own Internet company; apparently she's 'never seen anyone so IT literate' as me. I don't think so. I love computers, but I'm not better than anyone else. My Dad wanted me to take on his business, but I don't really fancy being an undertaker. I'm even more scared of death than I am of life. That's technically why I'm still alive. I don't think anyone would care if I died.

My parents have always preferred my sister. When I think of what I was like at her age, I wonder if we come from the same family. She's always out, has a million friends and, no doubt, changes boyfriends every five minutes. She's very pretty and wears a ton of makeup, which I've always found stupid since she has such a lovely face. I can imagine her talking to her friends: "Yeah, I have a sister, but she's so weird. There's nothing interesting about her; she has no life, no friends, and she's ugly and fat." It's probably what most people think, too. But see if I care! I decided a long time ago that I'd never let anyone upset me. I used to be walked over, trod on, made fun of. And why? You tell me. I've always minded my own business. I never tried to cause trouble. But somehow, it would always hit me in the face. At my very first day at school, when I was six, I was sitting on the pavement eating my lunch, and these two boys stood in front of me, whispering and giggling. I thought they were going to steal my food or beat me up, but after a moment, they disappeared behind me. Not long after, I could feel a hand on my rucksack. I knew exactly what was going on: my mother had put on it a big Care Bear sticker (the one with a rainbow on it – my favourite), and these boys were taking it off. But I didn't move. I was too scared. One of the boys then reappeared, shouting, "Look! I have a Care Bear sticker too!" And they laughed. I spent the whole afternoon crying, but no one noticed. I didn't tell anyone, not even my mother. What would have been the point? She'd probably have told me off for being a wimp. I've always thought I should deal with my problems by myself. Getting others involved would drag them into my suffering and possibly make things worse. That's why I've never had a proper boyfriend. I refuse to dump my load on somebody else. I was very fond of a boy once, when I was nineteen … but I made the mistake of being myself, telling him of my fears, my anger and bitterness. "It's too much for me", he said. "You need help". Me, need help? Ha! Since then, I decided I'd never get that close to anyone again. I haven't been with a man for over a year now, I don't need them. I certainly don't need love.

It's cold and grey outside; a real winter weather, except that it's summer. I hate winter. Sometimes, I dream of a long holiday on an island, just by myself. Somewhere warm and sunny, like Barbados. If I ever win the lottery, that's what I'll do. Or maybe I'll buy an island. So far I haven't been lucky; I've been playing for two years, every Wednesday and Saturday, but my numbers have never come out. I'd never give up though; because I know the day I don't buy a ticket will be the day that I miss the jackpot.

I have to go out. I'm standing at the bus stop, amongst a couple of old women and some school kids. I've only been out five minutes, and already I can tell that people are staring at me. They always do.

"Aren't you cold, dear?" asks one of the old women.

"No", I reply, shocked. So what if I am? Does she think I'm going to steal her coat or something? Yes, I am actually freezing in my short sleeve t-shirt, but why does she care? I refuse to wear warm clothes in summer, even if that means turning into an ice cube. It's the principle. I wish I had a car. I hate public transport. And I hate flashing my picture at the driver. I'm so ugly on it. I've never liked being photographed. When I was a child, my parents always had trouble trying to get me in the frame. I used to throw real tantrums. These days, I refuse to be photographed, which isn't too much of a problem since there aren't many occasions to take pictures anyway.

Today, I'm doing a double shift; I often do that, it's a good way to make more money. Plus, it's not like I have anything better to do with my time. Sometimes in the evening, Naomi comes around, or I go to hers. We watch videos, mostly. We both love Kevin Spacey. Secretly, I imagine myself tall, thin and gorgeous, and dancing mad dances with him, like Johnny and Baby in Dirty Dancing, until he whispers, "Come to bed, Melanie. I want to make love to you." If I ever told Naomi she'd laugh! She doesn't know the first thing about men though; she's never had a boyfriend. I don't know why, because she's quite pretty. But she says she wants to focus on her studies right now. I don't blame her, really. What's the point of being in a relationship, when you'll only end up hurt? I don't know how my parents do it. Maybe they're still together because it's convenient, with my sister and the house. I bet they don't even have sex anymore.

At lunchtime, Philip, my boss, asks to have a word. I know he's going to tell me off. Sooner or later, it was bound to happen. I don't know exactly what I've done, but it's been too long since the last time he had a go at me.

"Take a seat", he says as I enter his office.

"Don't look so mortified!" The grin on his face tells me he's going to enjoy every second of it. Sadistic bastard.

"You've been with us for quite some time, haven't you, Mel?"

"Well … yes."

"Do you ever think of moving forward?" I knew he'd try to get rid of me!

"No, I haven't given it much thought."

"The reason why I ask is that Paula, as you know, will be leaving us soon. Which means there will be a supervisor position available." He looks at me expectantly. "Do you see where I'm getting at?" He can't possibly mean what I think he's saying.

"I … don't know …"

"Would you like to be a supervisor, Melanie?" Surely he's not serious.

"Me?" He giggles.

"Yes, you. Why do you look so surprised? You are our best team member. You work hard, and you're very bright."

"Me?" I repeat. For a moment, he's silent. Then he adds, "If there was one thing I would change about you, it would be your self-confidence. Of course you can say no, but that would be a real shame. The job will involve mainly, as you probably know, evaluating the staff, writing them feedback and pretty much managing them. I honestly don't think you'd have any difficulties with that." I'm so, so shocked.

"Can ... Can I think about it?"

"Sure. Give me your answer by Monday." I leave his office slowly, feeling slightly uneasy. What should I do? A promotion! When I thought I'd get the sack!

"That's brilliant! I can't believe you haven't accepted yet!" Naomi shouts when I break the news to her after work.

"But, what if it doesn't work out? What if I can't do it?"

"Of course you can. You've been doing it for years."

"But I would have to tell people off!"

"So?"

"So, I can't do that."

"Mel, sooner or later, we all have to tell someone off. I bet you've told your sister off a million times!"

"It's not the same. And to be honest, I really don't do it that often anyway." She sighs. It's easy to tell she's losing patience.

"Well, it's your decision. But I don't see what you have to lose. If it doesn't work, you can always go back to being an operator." She doesn't understand. Go back to being an operator? How embarrassing would that be? Why did he ask me anyway? There are plenty of people who can do it better than me. But what will happen if I say no? I bet he'll sack me then! Oh God, what would I do? I can't do anything! I can imagine them. "That Melanie, what a loser! She can't even tell people off!" Maybe I should just not go back. I'd tell my parents they made me redundant or something. But then, I'd have to move back in with them and my sister would laugh at me. I have four days to make a decision. In four days, I'll either be a supervisor or unemployed. I open a bottle of red wine, pour myself a glass and sit on my bed. Naomi says I should get a sofa, but frankly, I'm not sure where I'd put it; my flat is very small. I don't actually know if you could call it a flat; more like a studio or a bed-sit. I have my own little kitchen, but I have to share the bathroom and toilets. That's all I can afford, you see. My parents don't like it much. They always worry about the neighbours and the area. Turnpike Lane isn't the best part of London, but obviously I can't live in Notting Hill.

Through the walls, I can hear shouting and cries. The neighbours upstairs always fight. I think they're both alcoholics. Once, they were so noisy that I had to call the police. I was so scared they'd know it was me that I didn't leave the flat for a week. I had to tell work I'd caught the flu. I decide to turn my computer on to distract myself. I don't often get emails, apart from the usual junk, but today I have one from Simon, a man from Virginia whom I met in a chat room. He's a nice guy, Simon. We have a lot in common. He works for an IT Consultancy, has two cats, and doesn't have many friends either. Once, we spent four hours online, talking about computers. After I've replied to his email, I go to a room called "PC Hell", where people seem to be having an argument about drivers and pilots. I love these kinds of discussions. I don't often take part in them, unless someone says something really stupid that I have to correct.

When I look at my watch it's gone three and as the screaming seems to have stopped, I go to bed. But like every night, I can't sleep. I haven't had a decent night of sleep for as long as I can remember. There's always so much going on in my head. I don't even know what it is, really. Just stuff. Like, why am I here? Why am I me? And what am I anyway? I'm not sure. I wonder if I'm the only one feeling like this. I mean, do people ever stop and think, why am I doing what I'm doing? Whenever I start thinking these things, I can't stop and tonight's no exception. So, as soon as I finally manage to close my eyes, the alarm goes off. I do the usual routine of having a shower, drinking coffee in front of GMTV, then getting ready and leaving for work. I spend most of the day observing Paula. She's so laid back ... I don't know how she does it. She shares jokes with everyone, she's on the phone to her friends all the time and when she evaluates people, it's as though she was giving them all a ten out of ten given how happy they look. I wonder how I would handle the job in her shoes. Philip said I was his best employee! Maybe Naomi's right; I should give it a go. I shouldn't dwell on what will happen if I fail. When I fail.

After my shift, I go to see Philip. When I tell him I've decided to take the job, a big smile appears on his face. Then a horrible thought comes to me. What if this is a plan to get rid of me? What if he gave me the job because he knew I wouldn't do it properly? That would be the best excuse for him to sack me!

"As of tomorrow, you'll be working alongside Paula", I hear him say. "She'll be pleased to train you." Pleased to show off, more like. She's never liked me. I sensed it ever since I started here. She's always been overly polite, and so fake. Somehow it didn't occur to me that she'd be training me. But what can I do? I can't exactly say to Philip, "Sorry, but I've changed my mind", or "I don't think I need any training", can I? Maybe I could call in sick; I could pretend I had an accident and broke my leg or something. By the time I'd recovered Paula would have left. And they might decide to take on someone else for the job! But what if they ask for a doctor's certificate? I don't know any doctors. Well, apart from my own, of course, but he'd get me arrested for fraud. I could make my father tell them I'm dead, I suppose.

When I get home, as there's nothing on TV, I decide to rent a video. It always takes me a while to pick one. It's like being in a sweet shop! Once I've chosen a couple of films, I head for the check out.

"Have you seen our offer, Madam? You can get a giant bag of crisps for £1, for every new release you rent. £2 for two bags", the clerk says as I'm about to pay.

"Oh, right. Well, OK then." I buy the two bags and head home. The thought of those crisps haunt me all the way. Did I make a mistake? Should I have only got one? I do feel quite hungry, but maybe crisps weren't the best thing to get. But I felt compelled to buy them. Forced, somehow. When I get in, I put the video machine on and sit on my bed with the bags of crisps. But I struggle to focus on the film; all my attention is concentrated on the crisps. I can't stop eating. One after the other, I put them in my mouth, chew and swallow, more and more quickly as the bag empties. Then I attack the second one. I can't tell if I'm still hungry or not. I just know I have to finish this bag off. It doesn't take me long to do so ... but as the last crisp disappears into my mouth I suddenly get an awful feeling of guilt. I shouldn't have done that. I'm so fat already! I hate it when that happens. I run to the toilet, lift the seat up and kneel down. Then, I put two fingers inside my mouth and sink them deep down my throat. I stay there for twenty, thirty minutes, until I'm sure there's nothing left inside me. My hands are red, swollen and covered in teeth bites; my face is flushed and my eyes are filled with water. You're so ugly, Melanie, I think, as I stare at my reflection in the mirror. But at least, you won't get fatter tonight! I wash my hands and face, clean the toilet and go back to my room. I re-wind the tape to the beginning, feeling much better.

****

"Is there anything you want to ask me about the training, Melanie?" Paula asks after our first shift together.

"No, no, I think I'm OK."

"Are you? You've been very quiet. Sure nothing's the matter?" What's it to her anyway?

"No, everything's fine, thanks." But she's still staring at me.

"Alright then. You've done very well today. I hope I can count you in for my leaving do?" Oh God. I hate leaving do's. Everyone getting drunk, loud and flirtatious with each other. It's so pathetic.

"I ... I'm not sure. When is it?"

"Friday the 18th."

"I … I think I'm away for the weekend. But I'll double check." Obviously that's a lie, but I could be, couldn't I? I have a life!

"Oh, OK. Well, I really hope you'll make it", she says with a big smile on her face. I know she's taking the piss out of me. She always does. It's like the time I wore this new jumper. When she saw me, I could tell she was trying hard not to laugh. She said something like "Oh, that's a really nice jumper" and asked me where I'd got it from. She even asked if I minded her getting the same one.

When I get home, the phone rings to tell me I have a message. It's from Naomi, asking me if I want to go to the pub.

"You should get a mobile", she announces as she hands me a glass of wine.

"I wouldn't have any use for it."

"People could get hold of you more easily."

"What people?"

"Well … me, for a start. And everyone else."

"But you don't have a mobile phone either."

"I'm actually planning to get one this weekend. You could come with me and get one too?"

"I really don't think there's much point. And they're too expensive anyway."

"Not all of them. You can get away with a decent £20 a month contract. That's not bad, is it?"

"That's £20 I could spend on something else."

"Like what?"

"I don't know ... wine or something."

"Well, you could always come with me though. You know about technical stuff, you could help me choose?" It's not like I have anything better to do anyway.

"If you like."

"By the way, that guy over there has been staring at you since we got here."

"What guy?"

"The one at the bar wearing a black shirt." When I look at him, he looks away, then his eyes meet mine again and he smiles.

"I think you've pulled!"

"He's not my type."

"What is your type?" I haven't thought about that in a long time.

"I don't know, not him."

"You always get men's attention. Everywhere we go! I don't believe you haven't seen at least one guy you fancied recently."

"I'm not interested. And I don't get that much attention. It's you they look at."

"No, it's not! I know when a guy fancies me. They make it quite obvious. And it's not as often as you."

"Even if it were true, which it isn't, I told you, I'm not interested." She looks around again, mumbles something and taps on her glass.

"What's it like?"

"What's what like?"

"You know ... it."

"IT? The film? Not that good. The book was much better."

"No, silly! I mean … sex." She blushes, and so do I, I think. I hate talking about sex.

"Oh. Well … I'm not the best person to ask."

"Why not? You've slept with men before. Did it hurt the first time?"
"Err …"

"Is it easy to have an orgasm? What's a blowjob like?"

"Stop it!" I hear myself shout maybe a bit too loud, as some people have turned around and are staring at me. "I meant … Sorry, I don't know. I don't want to talk about this anymore."

"Oh. Sure. Sorry." For a moment, we're both silent. As she empties her glass, I get up.

"Do you want the same?" She looks at me as though I'd told her I was becoming a man.

"Maybe we should just go."

"Oh. Are you sure?"

"Yes. I … I feel quite tired." I think I've offended her. I shouldn't have shouted. But I've apologised, haven't I? We leave and although she hugs me goodbye she still seems upset. She should know I hate talking about sex. I've told her enough times. She should just get herself some porn. And she'd learn everything she wants to learn. But knowing her, it'd probably put her off the whole thing. And so would listening to my own experiences.

On Saturday, I ended up buying a phone myself, just because she nags me to. We spend literally over two hours in the shop, Naomi going from one phone to another, asking me a mountain of questions.

"Do you think I should get a colour screen phone?" "Which one do you think is the prettiest?" "Should I get a flicky one?" "Oh, what do you think of this one?" She points at a square phone with a round screen.

"It looks like a washing machine." In the end, she buys one of the most expensive ones. I go for a cheaper version, but still I wonder if I'm doing the right thing. I mean, what do I need it for? If I'm not at work I'm usually in, so it's not like I can't be reached on my landline. But at least now Naomi will stop bugging me about it, so that's that.

"I think texting is the best invention ever", she says flicking through her manual as we leave the shop.

"Why is that?" I don't even know how it works.

"It's the quickest way to keep in touch! You don't even have to talk to people anymore."

"Sounds great." I can't believe it took me so long to get one. "Do you fancy a drink?"

"Now? But it's not even three!"

"So? It's Saturday, it's not like we have to work or anything." She looks hesitant. "I'll buy them."

"I guess we could go for one." We go to the nearest pub, "The Nag's Head", which is thankfully rather quiet. We sit at a table at the back, and on the ceiling in front of us is a screen playing music videos.

"So how's work been this week?" she asks after taking a sip of Diet Coke.

"You know. So-so", I say my eyes stuck to the screen. I hate all these blonde bimbos they constantly show you on TV these days. No talent whatsoever. I can't wait for the revival of music that actually means something.

"Really? Are you not enjoying being a supervisor?"

"I'm not sure."

"What is it?"

"I just hate the fact that Paula's always on my back."

"But … isn't she supposed to be?"

"It stresses me out. She watches everything I do, as if she didn't trust me or something."

"Has she said anything?"

"She doesn't need to. She keeps going on about what a good job I do, but if I really did she wouldn't be behind me all the bloody time, would she?"

"Maybe you should talk to her."

"What good would that do?"

"Well … Obviously it would depend on what you said. If you just asked her to fuck off she might not appreciate that. But you could tell her you're worried you're doing something wrong or you could even ask her if you could spend an hour on your own to see if you can manage. But to be honest, it's only been a week; she probably just wanted to make sure she'd taught you everything."

"I guess you're right. But I know she doesn't like me anyway."

"What makes you think that?"

"Everything. She pretends she's all nice and friendly but I can tell she's two-faced."

"But what has she done?"

"It's … just a vibe I got."

"A vibe. I think you're a bit paranoid."

"How can you say that? You haven't even met her!" I hate it when she uses that word.

"I know, but you do tend to think that people don't like you."

"Only if people actually don't."

"Name them."

"I … I don't know, everyone!" She bites her lip. I shouldn't have said anything. I knew she wouldn't understand.

"Do you want the same or something a bit more interesting?" I ask in an attempt to change the subject.

"I'm … I'm alright, actually."

"But your glass is empty."

"I know. But it's still quite early for something 'a bit more exciting'."

"Fine, have another soda then. I'll get you a proper drink on the next round." She sighs.

"OK, I'll have a lemonade then." When I come back with her soda and my wine, she frowns.

"Melanie, are you OK?"

"What do you mean?"

"I mean … how are you feeling these days?"

"How am I feeling? I'm not with you."

"I'm worried about you."

"Why?"

"Because you seem … I just …"

"If there's something on your mind just spit it out."

"Have you ever considered seeing a counsellor?" I'm baffled. I've heard a lot of stupid things coming from that woman, but this beats them all.

"A counsellor? What are you on about?"

"Just … Forget I mentioned it."

"What do you mean, a counsellor? Do you think there's something wrong with me?" I feel my face going warm.

"No! Not … something wrong … Just … a few things you might find helpful talking to someone about."

"Like what?"

"Like, when you say that you feel like you're in a dream and things aren't real, and you have to pinch yourself to make sure you're awake."

"So? I'm sure most people get that."

"I … don't think they do, actually. I know I don't."

"Well, you're not everyone, are you?"

"No, but I'd never heard of that before. And also, there's the fact that you think everyone is against you. And …"

"I don't think everyone's against me!" I interrupt.

"OK, I'll rephrase it then. That people don't like you very much. And I think you might have a bit of a drinking problem." I'm thrown. How dare she?

"I … don't know what you're talking about."

"Mel … I'm only saying this because I care about you."

"Yeah? Well it doesn't seem like it to me! Why don't you just mind your own business?" I down my wine, get up and run to the door.

"Melanie! Don't be silly! Please come back!"

"Leave me alone! I don't have problems; I don't need anybody's help!" I hear myself cry.

Once I leave the pub I keep on running until I'm totally out of breath and I'm sure she's not behind me anymore. I can't believe what she said. Telling me I have problems. Ha! Take a look at yourself, girl, I'm not the one who's still a virgin at twenty-one!

****

Four days have passed but I can't stop thinking about it. She was unreasonable. She had no right to talk to me like that. We haven't spoken since then. She tried to call me a few times but I didn't pick up. What would be the point? She's just like everyone else. Well, it doesn't matter. I can live without her. But now there's even less point having that stupid phone. It seems like she's given up trying to ring me; today she only sent me a text in the morning, and I haven't heard from her since then. What kind of friend is she if she can't make the effort of trying to patch things up? I don't see why I should bother if she doesn't. I decide to email Simon; he's about the only person left whom I don't want to kill right now. I tell him about work, what happened with Naomi and a number of random things I have on my mind. I know he doesn't mind me rambling. Then I go to the corner shop, and treat myself to a jar of gherkins. I just love them … they're filling, not fattening, and I like the acidic feeling I get in my stomach when I eat them. But for some reason, I can't manage to open the jar. I fiddle with it for about half an hour, using a knife to lift the lid off and running it under hot water, but nothing works. So I end up getting a hammer, thinking I could break the lid… But the whole thing smashes, covering my floor in vinegar, glass and bits of gherkin! I pick everything up, clean the carpet as much as I can and to make myself feel better, I end up back at the corner shop and buy a box of Jaffa cakes. Then it occurs to me that I could have just brought the jar back and asked them to open it themselves. Why does my brain only work when it feels like it?

Just as I was finishing the box of Jaffa cakes, my mother rings to tell me about Jenny's birthday in a couple of weeks.

"Have you thought of what to get her?"

"Money probably. Isn't that what she always asks for?"

"But it's so impersonal."

"But if that's what she wants, I don't see the problem. At least she'll spend it on whatever she likes."

"But what about clothes? She likes clothes."

"Have you actually seen her wear any of the clothes you've bought her?"

"Well … yes, I'm sure she has. Two days ago she wore the black and red jumper I got her for Christmas."

"Yes, but she chose it, didn't she?"

"Are you saying she doesn't like my presents?" She asks after a long pause. She's always so touchy when it comes to Jenny.

"I'm not saying that, I just think she might appreciate money more."

"Oh."

"Why don't you take her out and buy her something then?"

"That's a good idea. But I won't have time before her birthday, what with the shop and all." My mother runs a charity shop and she always talks about it as if it were Harvey bloody Nichols. "Maybe you could take her?"

"Me?" She can't be serious. It's always such a hassle to get there.

"Well, yes, I know she'd be pleased to spend some time with you."

"I don't see why."

"Because you're sisters! You used to be so close when you were younger." I don't know where she got that from. My mother has always imagined us as the perfect family, all of us being like best friends. She watches too many American films.

"So will you do it?" I can't think of anything worse. But if I said no she would never forgive me.

"I can't spend too long with her. I'm really busy."

"Of course, I completely understand Darling. I'm sure she'll be looking forward to it."

****

"Hey Mel, how are you?" Jenny asks as she opens her bedroom door. I hadn't seen inside her room since I moved out. The walls are covered with posters of boy-bands but the floor and surfaces are as tidy and clean as they used to be. I bet my mother still does it all for her.

"I'm fine, thanks. Ready?"

"Yeah! Thanks so much for talking to mum. I don't think I could have handled another woolly jumper. "

"That's OK. So where do you want to go?"

"Could we go to the shopping centre?" I hate shopping centres.

"Sure."

"There's this jacket my mate Hannah's got from H&M, and it's just fab!"

"You want the same jacket as your friend?" Teenagers are so common. At her age, I refused to wear anything I saw on someone else. It did make it quite difficult to buy clothes sometimes.

"No, but I want to check out the shop. I don't get the chance to go there too often, since mum and dad are always too busy."

"Can't your friends take you?"

"None of them drive yet."

"You could always take the bus, like we're doing now."

"I guess so. But my friends prefer hanging out in bars."

"In bars? At your age?"

"Well … Yeah. I look older than my age. Not that I drink or anything …"

The centre is packed with people; Jenny wanders from one shop to another, looking at every possible thing. She probably knows how much I resent this and is just doing it to annoy me.

"There it is!" She shouts pointing at the H&M sign. Again, she looks at everything in the shop, even men's clothes.

"What are you looking at these for? You wear men's clothes now?"

"Err … no, no. I … I was just curious."

"Anything you like here?" I ask, trying to make her hurry.

"I can't decide. There's too much choice! What do you think?" She asks as she picks what looks more like a belt than a skirt.

"It's … very short."

"Oh. What about this then?" She points at the same skirt but about two inches longer. "Still too short?"

"If you like it, it doesn't matter what I think."

"Of course it does. If you think I'll look stupid in it I don't want it." Tarty would be a better word.

Twenty minutes later, once she's decided to go for a black top and some denim trousers (on my advice), I take her for a coffee. She didn't seem ready to go home yet, so I figured if we had to spend more together we may as well do it sitting down.

"So how's work going?"

"It's fine."

"Mum said you got promoted?"

"Yeah."

"That's great! I can't wait to get a job. Get out of the house." No doubt my mother would be devastated if she knew. I don't blame her, though.

"I didn't think you got too much of a hard time there."

"Oh, I really hate it! You're so lucky, living in London."

"It's not that great. Just more people. And louder."

"Exactly. It's so boring here", she says a frown on her face. "I was wondering … Could I come and spend some time at your flat?"

"My flat? Why?"

"Because … It'd be nice to go to London. And to spend some time with you, because you don't come down very often." Why would she want to spend time with me? I bet she just wants to use the flat, just because I live in London. I'm not a damn hotel, am I? "Will you come for my birthday? I'm inviting some mates over and then we're going clubbing. But don't tell mum and dad, they think we're going to my friend Laura's!"

"You go clubbing as well?" Have all the bouncers in England gone blind or something?

"I've never been, but Sarah's given me a fake ID. Don't tell anyone though!"

"Oh. Well, I don't know, I think I'm working that day."

"You could come afterwards … Surely they don't make you work at night, do they?" I can't think of anything worse than being stuck somewhere full of spotty and arrogant teenagers.

"I'll have to see." She stares at her empty cup and bites her lips.

"Mel?"

"What?"

"Have you ever … taken drugs?"

"Drugs? No, never. Only stupid, sad people take drugs. And anyone who says differently is an idiot."

"Right. Sure. So, will you come? Please?"

"I'll try. Are you done with your drink? I've got a few things I need to sort out before the end of the day." I make the mistake of walking her to the house and when she opens the front door, my mother appears. Even though I point out that I'm in a rush, I'm forced to have tea with her and listen to her rambling about the shop, and how she might have to hire someone new "because it's getting really busy, but it's really hard to trust someone you don't know these days", which makes me think she's implying I should go for the job, but I pretend I don't take the hint. When I finally manage to get home, I turn my computer on.

Hey Mel,

Sorry you're feeling so down. I'm not sure what to say about your friend; maybe she was just trying to help? Seems to me like she cares, but I know friends don't always say the right thing at the right time. Maybe you should try to talk to her though; she probably feels really upset too.

On a happier note, I have good news: I'm coming over to London in a few weeks for some business and it would be a great opportunity to finally meet up! I don't know the exact dates, but as soon as I do I'll let you know.

Take care,

Simon x

He's coming over. He wants to meet me! What am I going to do? I have to ring Naomi and tell her. But I'm not technically talking to her. Maybe Simon's right; maybe she was trying to help. She shouldn't have said what she said, but she did apologise. I pick up the phone and dial her number, feeling a slight pinch in my stomach.

"Hello?"

"Nam? It's Mel."

"Mel? Oh, hi. How are you? It's…been a while."

"Yeah, I know."

"I'm sorry about everything."

"Let's just forget about it. Guess what? Simon's coming to London and he wants to see me!"

"Oh my God! That's brilliant!"

"No, it's not! It's really scary."

"Why? From what you've said he seems really nice."

"He is. But it's one thing having a pen friend, and another meeting them in the flesh."

"What have you got to lose?"

"What if he doesn't like me? What if he thinks I'm stupid or something?"

"I don't see why he would. And even if he does, you won't have to see him ever again anyway."

The more we talk about it, the more I want to meet him. He seems like a very nice person. Maybe we would become good friends. Great friends. I mean, there's bound to be at least one person in this world that I can get on with, right?

Chapter 2

I was thinking I could take him to the London Eye. He'd probably like that, wouldn't he? Most tourists do. And he said he liked Italian food, so we could go to Fernando's in Soho. It's not expensive and their wine is delicious. And maybe we could see a film at the cinema, and then take a walk along the river! OK, so I'm getting carried away. And probably being stupid. But we get on so well online, there's no reason why we wouldn't in real life. Anyway, Paula only has only a few days left and she hasn't been bothering me much lately. She said I should try to work by myself as much as possible because soon she wouldn't be there to help me anymore. As if I need her help! She spends more time chatting than doing any work. I had to give ten pounds for her leaving present. Ten pounds! They said it wasn't compulsory but everyone else had done it, so I couldn't say no, could I? It's going to be a very expensive present, that's all I can say. I bet they wouldn't bother if I left. I couldn't imagine anyone spending ten pounds on me. And they'd probably throw a party once I'm gone! So many things are happening: Jenny's party, Paula's leaving do on Friday, and of course, Simon. I don't know how I will cope with all this. I have to prioritise: I should concentrate on Simon. Jenny's sixteen, and she'll have dozens of friends coming to her party, so she won't notice if I'm not there. And she'll have probably forgotten she's invited me anyway. Same for Paula. Plus I'll never see her again after the 18th, so it doesn't matter.

I wonder what Simon looks like. I've never asked him. I've thought about it more than once, but I don't want him to think I'm interested in him in that way, because I'm not. I mean, I've thought about us falling in love before, but that was just make believe. Although he said he didn't have a girlfriend. Not that I care, but it's good to know. Having said that, I wonder why. Maybe he's unattractive. That would make sense. Attractive men have tons of girlfriends. Because that's what people want, isn't it? Someone they fancy. Not someone who's nice, or caring, but someone they can shag. That's why she's single, I bet you think. Yep. But I'm not particularly nice or caring anyway.

****

Hey Mel,

I've got the dates: 21st till 3rd. Thanks for your offer to pick me up from the airport, but I'll have a taxi waiting. I'm going to be pretty busy 'til the weekend; maybe we could do lunch on Saturday? But there's plenty of time to arrange it.

Simon

Wow. That's much sooner than I thought. But I don't know why I'm nervous really; it's only lunch, right? Just two people having food somewhere. I have to eat a salad. I can't have him think I'm a greedy pig. Oh God, I'm so fat. And what am I going to wear? I hate all my clothes!

"Why don't you borrow something of mine?" Naomi suggests. Because your clothes are hideous, is what I want to reply.

"You know I hate pink."

"Not all of my clothes are pink!" She opens the doors of her cupboard, picks up a couple of items and hands them to me. It's a skinny white top and a long black skirt.

"I'm too fat for those."

"Are you mad? They're size 10! They'll fit you just fine."

"What if they don't?"

"If they don't, you'll try something else on. Or, we could do that thing you resent so much ..."

"Don't say it."

"But we don't have to go anywhere big!"

"I'd rather look on the internet."

"I know; but you do realise that most of the clothes you bought from the internet never fit you."

"That's not true."

"Of course it is. You swim in everything you own! At least let me look with you."

"Whatever."

"We haven't got much time. He's coming over in a few days, right?"

"Yep."

"Well you'd better make an effort then! Maybe we could check out some shops this weekend?" She sounds so excited you'd think she was the one meeting him.

"Not this weekend. I feel too fat to look at anything." She gives me a look somewhere between outrage and disbelief.

"Have you actually eaten today?"

"Of course I've eaten."

"What did you have?"

"What kind of question is that?" She knows I hate talking about food.

"A sensible one."

"Who are you, the food Gestapo?" She raises her eyebrows and sighs. I don't think she should be the one getting moody. She's been such an interfering cow lately.

"Anyway, are you going to your boss's leaving do tomorrow?"

"No. I'll tell them I've got a headache or something." I'm a very good liar. I enjoy lying; it gives me a sense of control. Once when I was twelve, I went into a corner shop and told the owner my dog had just died. I cried so much even the most heartless person would have fallen for it. The man looked so alarmed! He gave me a bottle of strawberry milkshake and a chocolate bar. I was such a pig at that age. I've lied for as long as I can remember; although I don't do it as much as I used to. There's hardly anyone to lie to, these days. I'm honest most of the time, unless people start asking personal questions. So the next day, I arrive at work with a box of Paracetamol, and make sure everyone sees when I take some.

"Are you OK?" Paula asks eventually. I put on my most miserable face and moan my reply.

"Not really ... I've had a headache since last night. If it doesn't go away, I'll have to pass on tonight I'm afraid."

"Oh, sure. There'll be plenty more occasions. Anyway, I'll be in touch with everyone." Oh joy. Well, at least I'm all clear for tonight. Except that by five I've taken so many tablets that I'm completely drowsy and ready to pass out on my desk. Everyone spends the whole day in an annoyingly happy mood. The thought of free drinks always has that effect on them; it makes them act even more stupidly than usual.

I get back to the flat planning a quiet night in, with a video and some wine; but as soon as I have turned the TV on and sat down I hear my neighbour scream. As usual, I turn the volume up, and try to drown the noise with Eastenders. I don't even like it, but if I started watching a film now I'd be too distracted by the arguments to concentrate. Most of the time, they give in after half an hour, so hopefully I won't have too long to wait. Except that when Eastenders finishes, they're still at it. It actually sounds even louder and more violent than when it started. I can almost hear every word they're saying.

"Who the fuck do you think you are?"

"I've had enough of this, it's over!"

"It's not over until I fucking say it is! You get that?"

"Let go of me!"

"Where do you think you're going?"

Part of me thinks I should maybe do something; but then, they always argue. And what could I do anyway? Then I hear a door slam. And then, I jump. Someone is knocking on my door. It's her. Who else would it be? Why the hell is she knocking on my door? Oh God, I can't let her in. If I do, he'll be here next, and I'll be the one in trouble. I quickly cut off the sound of the TV. Please go away. Please go away.

"Hello? Hello?" It is her. Why is this happening to me?

"There you are." His voice echoes, as though there were ten of him. He's on my doorstep too.

"Leave me alone!"

"Come back and we'll talk this through. I'm sorry I shouted at you."

"I don't want to go back in there. Never!"

"Am I going to have to force you?"

"Fuck you! Argh! You're hurting me! Let go!" The voice fades gradually, and then the door upstairs slams again. Then there's another noise, like something falling on the floor, and then nothing. I really should complain to the Council. I'm so fed up with this shit. I can't believe she tried to involve me in it. Why is she staying with this arsehole anyway? It's obvious he's deranged. I damn hope it's over for tonight; I'm shaking all over.

Thankfully it's the last I hear from them, and with the Paracetamol still doing its job, for once I get a decent night of sleep. Work is quiet the next day; most people are usually off at weekends, and the few that are here are hungover from Paula's party anyway. Last night's events had made me forget that from today on, I'm a supervisor. It goes well: I don't have to shout at anyone and I get no complaints from the people interviewed. No one ever complained about me but I know some people get into a lot of trouble because they said the wrong thing, like the guy who, when interviewed, said he was fifteen when he left school, and the interviewer laughed and said "Really?" On the way back home I feel slightly uplifted. That is until I reach my block and find four police cars outside. There are people everywhere and an officer is standing by the main door.

"Excuse me, can you tell me what's happened?" I don't particularly enjoy talking to policemen, but it's not everyday I see them around my house.

"Do you live here, madam?"

"Yes."

"Can you tell me what number?"

"Three."

"I'm afraid one of your neighbours was found dead this afternoon. Miss Cartwright." Oh God. Oh no. "Are you OK? Do you need to sit down?" He grabs my arm and helps me sit on the pavement. My head is spinning, my heart beating so hard it might explode. He killed her. The noise I heard yesterday. Something falling on the floor. Then, there was nothing. It was her.

"Did you know Miss Cartwright well, madam?"

"Err … No, not really. Who … How did you find her?"

"A friend of hers came here after Miss Cartwright failed to turn up at her house; she tried to call her but Miss Cartwright never picked up. She knocked on the door but as there was no answer she called her mobile again and heard it ring inside. Apparently Miss Cartwright had a somewhat violent relationship with the man she lived with, so he suspected something was wrong and rang us. When we got here we found Miss Cartwright lying on the floor. She had died a few hours earlier. It seems she was hit with a heavy object. Sorry, madam, I don't know your name?"

"Melanie. Stevens."

"Ms Stevens, did you hear anything suspicious last night? An argument, shouting, a fight? Ms Stevens?"

"No. I … I fell asleep. Early. I had taken a lot of Paracetamol because I had a headache. So … I fell asleep."

"I see. We're looking for the man, her boyfriend. Do you have any idea where he could have gone?"

"No. I ... I've never really spoken to him."

"Alright. Well, let me give you our number; if you can think of anything that might be of help to us, please, do call. Thank you for your time, Ms Stevens."

I killed her. She knocked on my door. She needed my help. That's so horrible. She didn't deserve to die. Could I go to prison? Oh God. I didn't know he was going to do that, did I? They can't prove anything. I stayed in, I didn't make any noise. The TV. The bloody TV. But it wasn't that loud. No, it wasn't; I could still hear them fight over the sound. And I could have easily fallen asleep with it still on. Maybe I should tell the police. I could always say I'd forgotten. I need to ask Nam's advice.

"I don't think you should get involved. It seems pretty obvious to them he did it anyway, so I would stay out of it."

"But I feel so bad."

"Don't blame yourself. If it hadn't happened last night it would have happened some other time."

"But she said she'd leave him. I heard her. She wanted to go."

"Hadn't they been there like a million times before?"

"I guess."

"Honestly, Mel, don't worry. I'm sure they'll catch him", she says calmly. She baffles me sometimes. Someone has just died. She got killed because her boyfriend was a bully. I thought by keeping away from the news I was safe from a lot of shit; I never imagined anything like this could happen in my own building. The world is a really sick place. "Anyway, I've got some really exciting news!" Usually, when she says that, she's either passed an exam or lost a couple of pounds. Not that I'm not interested, but the first reminds me how uneducated I am, and the latter, that I'm fat.

"What is it?" I ask trying to sound enthusiastic.

"I have a date!"

"You ... what?"

"I have a date!" She repeats. That's what I'd heard the first time but I thought it couldn't be right.

"What do you mean, you have a date?"

"With a man!" If I weren't sitting I'd collapse.

"I ... don't understand."

"This guy in my course called George ... we've been talking quite a lot lately, and this morning, he asked me if I wanted to go for a drink with him tomorrow night."

"But ... you don't go out with men."

"He's really cute! I still can't believe it!"

"But ... what about your studies?"

"Yeah, well, one drink isn't going to kill me, is it? I'm so nervous! My first date ever!" I don't know whether to laugh or cry. She doesn't know anything about men. What on earth will they talk about? "Are you still there?"

"What? Yes. I'm just ... surprised."

"Not as much as I am! What do you think I should wear? What about my little black dress?"

"Well ... You should wear trousers. A dress is ... too revealing. You don't want him thinking you're easy."

"Right."

"And a jumper. Or something with long sleeves."

"But it's summer! I'll die. I'll be all sweaty and he'll freak out!"

"A polo shirt then."

"Mel! I'm going on a date, not to a rugby match! Are you trying to make me look as unattractive as possible or something?"

"Don't be stupid! You asked my opinion and I'm giving it to you. If you want to look like a tart, it's your problem, but I'm not the one you should talk to." That probably sounded a bit harsh, but the words just came out. For a moment, she doesn't say anything.

"Do you know what I think? I think you're jealous."

"Jealous? Of what?"

"Of me having a date."

"That's ridiculous."

"Then why are you being so unfair?"

"I'm not being unfair. I told you, I just don't want him to get the wrong impression of you."

"But I wasn't trying to look like a tart. I just wanted to look nice!" I know I have to lie now.

"I'm sorry. I didn't mean to offend you. If you want to wear a dress, I think the black one will be the nicest."

"Really?"

"Yeah."

"Thanks. I'll let you know all about it!" I don't want to know about it. I don't want to hear about how great her evening was. But it's bound to go wrong. It has to.

At 10:30 the next evening, I get a text message from Naomi. "Mel, I'm in the bar's toilet; he's asked me 2 go back 2 his place! What should I do? Please reply quickly, I can't hide here 4ever!"

I decide to ignore it. She's big enough to know what she wants. And she wouldn't like my answer anyway. And I hate the way she writes her texts; she's too lazy to spell properly! I bet she's going home with him. Tart! But what do I care anyway? If she wants to get off with the first man she meets it's her problem. I don't see why she always asks my opinion when she never listens to it anyway. Then she wonders why I get upset! And I bet she'll never call. She's replaced me now.

An hour later, the phone rings. At this time, it can only be her. As I don't pick up she calls my mobile. Why is she bothering me now? Maybe she's in his bathroom and wants to know how to give him a blowjob. But surprisingly enough, her voicemail says she's at home. She wants me to call her back but I'm really not in the mood. I don't care if she's had a nice evening. I don't care if he's the man of her bloody life!

****

I'm starting to miss Paula. Well, not so much her than the fact that when she was here, people left me in peace. Now everyone's asking me questions. I even have to go and talk to them if they have problems. And if someone is taking too long a break, I have to tell them off. It's like being at school again! Plus I spend the whole day worrying about whether it's safe for me to go back to the flat. What if her boyfriend comes back for me? He knows she came to me for help. But he must realise people are looking for him. On the other hand, if he did kill me, he'd do me a bloody good favour. When I'm back at the flat, I somehow find myself waiting for him, thinking of the way he might finish me off. It would have to be quick; I don't want a long death. I don't want to be aware that I'm dying. He could hit me, like he did with her. I wonder what he used. A big ornament? A frying pan? And I wonder who'd come to my funeral. Maybe I'd be in the papers: "Killer boyfriend comes back for his neighbour." The people who knew me would say, "What a shame, she seemed like such a nice girl. I wish I'd got to know her better."

"Melanie, Carl was late again this morning. I think you should let him know." Damn Phil. Can't he do his dirty work himself? I don't even know Carl; I hardly ever say hello to him. I really don't want to do this but if I don't do it now I'll get told off, so I walk towards him, rehearsing in my head what I'm going to say.

"Hi, Carl."

"Hi."

"You were late this morning."

"Yeah?" He stares at me and I understand that I'm not going to get much more out of him.

"Can you tell me why?"

"My train was delayed."

"Right. Well... Can you make sure it doesn't happen again?"

"Unfortunately, I don't have magical powers; but if I did, I'd certainly make all the trains in the world arrive on time." I wonder how much trouble I'd get in if I punched him.

"I appreciate that, but you could just get an earlier train maybe?"

"Then I'd have to leave half an hour early, which means that I'd have to get up half an hour early."

"That's not my problem. You can't be late all the time."

"I don't get paid enough to get up half an hour earlier!" He's doing it on purpose. He's blatantly trying to piss me off.

"Look, if you don't like it, you can always look for another job!" To this he mumbles something and puts his headphones back on.

"Melanie, can I have a word?" I hadn't noticed Phil standing behind me. I get the feeling he's not going to congratulate me. "What happened with Carl?" I don't see why he's asking, he's probably heard the whole conversation. And what was he doing listening to me in the first place? "When you need to tell someone off, can you take them on the side, in my office or somewhere empty, because otherwise the people on the other end of the phone will hear it, and it doesn't give out a very professional image of the company." Not very professional. What about the way he spoke to me? Do people talk to their superior like that? And then I get told off because the kitchen is a mess. Am I supposed to be the cleaner as well now? On my break I get another message from Naomi. I don't particularly want to talk to her, but I'd do anything to take my mind off work for a few minutes.

"Took you long enough."

"Yeah, sorry. I fell asleep early last night."

"You? Sleep?"

"Yes. I was very tired."

"Aren't you going to ask me how it went?"

"How what went?"

"My night, silly!"

"Go on, then."

"Well, it was great. We went for a drink in this tiny pub off Goswell Road, then he took me for dinner in an Indian restaurant, and then we went to another pub. He's such a nice guy. We talked for hours."

"But you didn't go to his place?"

"No. I wanted to take it slowly. But we kissed loads!" Yuck.

"Right."

"Aren't you happy for me?"

"That's ... great. So what now?"

"I'm seeing him again tomorrow night."

"That's ... great."

"I know, you keep saying! Maybe you could meet him soon?"

"Err ... maybe, yes."

"He's really lovely. I think you'll like him." I try hard not to laugh. Why on earth would I like him?

"Maybe we could all have dinner sometime? Or just go for a drink or something."

"Yeah, maybe. But let's see how things go first. You've only been out with him once."

"I know. I'm sorry, I'm just so excited!" I don't see why. He's probably stupid, ugly and he'll dump her as soon as he's slept with her. But she needs to make her own mistakes. I didn't like my first time. It was fast, painful and tasteless. I'd only known the guy for a week or so; I was camping with my mother, dad, Jenny and my uncle Patrick and my aunt Di and I'd find him at the site's bar every night. Once, we got very drunk together and I ended up in his tent. It went so fast it took me a while to realise what was going on. He sounded so surprised when I asked him what he was doing! He told me he'd stop if I wanted him to, but I didn't. I just wanted to get it over and done with. I don't regret it; if it hadn't happened that night it would have happened later and it would have been the same anyway, no matter who it was with. I hate being touched. I hate feeling someone else's skin on mine. I don't think many men would get pleasure from me I've not got any to give.

Chapter 3

Whenever I speak to Naomi, all I hear about is George. Apparently, he's "handsome, kind and funny". He takes her places, even cooks for her. She says she's never been this happy. She's known him five minutes and already he's the best thing since sliced bread. If I spoke half as much about Simon as she does about him, she would have died of boredom a long time ago. I haven't seen her since before her first date. She did ask me out, but I didn't see the point since all I was going to hear all night was how lovely he was. I was planning to drag her to Jenny's party but I doubt she'll want to now. One more reason for me not to go either. I never got invited to parties when I was her age. The only ones I went to were school ones, when they were compulsory. There was a disco once, at the end of a school trip to Scotland and when the ballads came on, no one had invited me to dance, so I ended up with my Geography teacher. Not that I wanted to, but I felt obliged to accept when he offered. I was quite drunk then, otherwise I'd never have done it. Obviously after that everyone made fun of me. For the rest of the year they kept making jokes, and someone even said I was expecting his child.

At the time I didn't realise, but now it's clear he knew what he was doing; he just wanted to ridicule me. And I didn't even get good grades out of it! I can't imagine being pregnant. It must feel so strange, having something living inside you. Like in 'Alien'. I don't think I'd make a good mother anyway. I'd hardly have any money to look after a kid, and no patience whatsoever. I'd be like most parents these days shouting at them all the time. God knows why they have children. And even if you are a nice parent, chances are they'll grow up to be total bastards only calling when they need money and when you're old enough they'll put you in a home, waiting impatiently for your death to get their inheritance. Naomi loves children. She wants three, apparently. She's probably already thinking of having them with George. I wonder what her kids will look like. I wonder what my kids would look like. I don't look like my parents; Jenny does. I'm sure I was adopted. I was found under a rock or in one of these wheelie bins you find outside supermarkets. When they saw me there, they just felt obliged to take me home. Christian Aid, that sort of thing. I used to go to church every Sunday when I was young; I hated it. All these people there who felt they were good because they prayed and thanked the Lord but behaved like arseholes for the rest of the week. The good people are the non-believers. The ones that act out of kindness and not because they think that if they don't they'll be punished. People want to believe they'll go to heaven because they can't stand the idea that there is nothing after death. And as to reincarnation. I think I'd rather go to hell than come back to this place. Or maybe this is it. This is where people who behaved badly end up after life. It makes sense, doesn't it?

****

It's raining today. The heavy, stormy type of rain that soaks you. I love that. I love the feeling of water running down my face. I love the smell of rain. I love seeing people running, trying to escape from it. The streets are so quiet when it rains. I'm seeing Naomi tonight. For some insane reason I've agreed to meet George. We are going to his favourite restaurant apparently ("Surely if he is as nice as you claim him to be, he would have let you choose?" I wanted to say), somewhere called La Mesange, on New Bond Street. I must say I'm nervous. I don't know why. Maybe I'm scared I might like him. But what are the odds? Anyway, I'm going there with an open mind and I've decided to give the poor sod a chance. I arrive late, as I refuse to be the first one there and have to sit at the table by myself, looking like a loser. I'm greeted by a tall, blond, slimy pin-up guy, who shakes my hand and introduces himself as "George, Naomi's boyfriend." No shit, if he hadn't said anything I wouldn't have guessed.

"Sorry I'm late", I throw in casually.

"That's OK!" Naomi cries. She sounds something between hysterical and anxious. As I sit down the waiter comes and hands me a menu. I order a glass of wine and start looking for the salads. I scan the pages quickly at first, then start again more slowly, and soon realise to my horror that there are no salads on this menu. I don't think I've ever been anywhere that didn't sell salads. What kind of place is this?

"What are you having, Mel? The salmon seems quite nice."

"I … can't seem to find any salads."

"Oh no, they don't have those here. They're a bit too eclectic for salads!" I can't believe Naomi took me somewhere that doesn't sell salads. She's only known me for fifteen years!

"Their chicken is really tasty", the pin-up man adds.

"Have you chosen?" The waiter asks when he comes back with my drink.

"I'll take the salmon. Number 46."

"And I'll take 51."

"Do you have anything light?" I restrained myself from saying "normal".

"Light?"

"Yes, light. As in, not fattening."

"Well … I'm not sure, let me think."

"Can you just make me a plate of vegetables?"

"A plate of vegetables?" The waiter repeats. I'm starting to think I'm talking Chinese.

"Yes. You know carrots, tomatoes, peas, etc?"

"Err …" Now he looks in pain, as if I'd asked him to do a roly poly in the middle of the restaurant.

"I … I will be back." And off he goes.

"You've given him grief!" Naomi laughs.

"I didn't realise vegetables could be such hard work."

"I think he's just not used to people asking him questions!" The boyfriend says.

"But surely, that's his job?" They give each other a quick glance.

"I'm sure they'll find you something", Naomi says in a reassuring tone.

"So, Melanie, Naomi tells me you work in Market Research?"

"Yes."

"Do you enjoy it?"

"You know. It's a job, really. Pays the rent, buys the food, that sort of thing."

"Sure."

"Melanie loves computers! I always tell her she should work in IT!"

"Is that so?" George asks. Why is he pretending to care?

"Well, computers are part of everyone's life now. People who don't know how to use them should really start learning or they'll soon be left behind, if they aren't already."

George comes back "Oh, I think I'm quite safe there, being a lawyer doesn't require a large amount of computer literacy, if you have a PA!"

How typical of men. I don't know why they don't just call their PAs "whores".

"George wants to be a human rights lawyer. Isn't that exciting?" Naomi throws in.

"Trust me, computers are essential", I say ignoring her. "And you can't expect someone else to do all the work for you." It amuses me, seeing him so helpless and uncomfortable after everything I say. A part of me is expecting him to jump out of his seat and run away. But he doesn't; he manages to keep calm, patient and polite up until the end. They both seem extremely relieved when our plates arrive (the waiter never told me if I could be served my vegetables, but came back with a plate full of green beans and potatoes), and George doesn't open his mouth again until he's finished his dish. I barely touch mine: everything is covered in the greasiest sauce. I'm not remotely hungry anyway, the sight of these two is a real put-off. Naomi talks about her exams and how she's worried she might fail, and he tells her she's too clever not to pass. She complains about her weight and he assures her she's very thin; she mentions cutting her hair short and he says she's very attractive with long hair. It's all so sickening I struggle to keep the small amount of food I've eaten inside. Next thing he'll be singing under her balcony! At least the wine offers me a small consolation; I drink far more of it than them, but what the hell. I think Naomi's trying to be nice in front of him, because not once does she mention my weight, nor counselling, nor any of the "problems" she usually finds in me. After spending more than two hours in the restaurant (after the main course George ordered a dessert, so I had to endure another half hour there), we finally leave, and by that time I've drunk more wine than them two put together. George offers to take me back home but I decline, even though I'm struggling to remember where I actually live; I don't know how long it takes me to get back, but I'm so relieved I'm rid of them that I would have been happy if I'd spent the night on the pavement. Love is boring, I think to myself as I walk inside the flat. But it is fairly entertaining to see others use it as a way to find happiness. Good luck to them!

****

I've made my mind up: I won't go to Jenny's party. There's no point, I'd only be a burden to her. I've told my mother and she wasn't happy; but she doesn't understand Jenny anyway. She thinks she looks up to me and wants to be like me! I've told Jenny too and she said I could at least come for an hour or so and leave if I didn't like it, but I told her I'd feel too uncomfortable. I'd spend the whole time standing by myself like an idiot; I wouldn't have anything to talk to her friends about. She said she hoped I'd change my mind! She's sweet. But to be honest I've already planned my Saturday: Ghost, The Crying Game and two bottles of wine! I don't know what I'd do without my videos ... I'd love to have a big film collection. I really wish I'd win the Lottery. But then, if I did win, I'd probably lose my privacy; I'd have journalists taking pictures of me and asking me what I'm planning to do with the money. I couldn't deal with that! So in a way, it's a good thing I'm poor. But who knows, maybe Simon will prove me wrong about the human race, and we'll get married, and then I'll be able to afford all the films in the world! Only a few days left until he comes to London. It's a shame I'll have to wait more than a week to see him though; but maybe he'll find some spare time before that! Oh God, I'm becoming hysterical again. Maybe he won't find any time at all. But then, he did seem keen, didn't he? I should stop worrying. What will happen, will happen. He's not the type of person who would say something and do the opposite. But then, I've never met him; he could be a woman for all I know! Now that's a scary thought. I'd never even considered it before. No, that wouldn't happen. Men pretend to be women but women don't pretend to be men. What would be the point of lying since we're about to meet in the flesh? Maybe I should ask him to send me a picture. But then he'd ask for mine. And then he definitely wouldn't want to meet me! I guess I'll just have to trust him.

As I browse the video store once again, I feel content, although I'm not the only one who has decided to stay in tonight; thankfully I've found the two films I wanted, but before going home I have another look around, just because it keeps me outside for a while. Sometimes, it's nice to be somewhere else than the flat; not anywhere, of course, but here is perfect. When I get back I make myself a salad, get the wine out and rewind the films. Why do people never rewind the videos before giving them back? I always do. Maybe I should stop, since no one else bothers. By 11:30pm I've drunk most of my wine and the second film is almost finished. I am starting to feel tired, the wine being exceptionally strong; so I close my eyes and start to drift off, when my mobile rings. I don't recognise the number. I cut it off, telling myself it must be a mistake. And even if it weren't, who the hell rings someone at 11:30pm at night? Someone who is damn rude, that's who. Then it rings again. The same number flashes on the screen. It seems to be a house phone. I cut it off again, and turn my mobile off. If it's that bloody important they'll leave a message. I wonder if it's Naomi, calling me from George's house. But why would she do that? We haven't spoken since we went to the restaurant. Maybe she wanted to invite me over or something. But that seems as likely as me shagging the Prince of Wales. Curiosity taking over, the wine probably helping, I turn my phone back on and decided to call back, withholding my number. No one picks up. I ring again, and again, and finally someone answers.

"Hello?"

"Who's this?"

"Sorry?"

"Who are you? You've just rung my phone."

"I don't think it was me, dear. This is a payphone." I bet it was a prank call.

"Oh. Right. Where is this payphone located?"

"In a hospital."

"A hospital?" That's strange.

"That's right, dear."

"Did you see anyone using this phone? Just a minute ago?"

"Err … No, I wasn't paying attention. I just happened to walk past it when it rung."

"Is there anyone around you? Anyone who just sat down?"

"Yes, plenty. People are coming and going."

"What do they look like?"

"I beg your pardon?"

"The people! What do they look like?"

"I'm sorry darling; I don't have time for games."

"No, wait! I need to know who's just called me!" But the line goes dead. Bastard! Who the hell could have called me from a hospital? And why aren't they calling back? But it can't be too serious, no, it can't be, or they would have left a message. God, I wish I hadn't drunk so much wine, I can't think straight right now. OK, who do I know who's likely to be in a hospital? What a stupid question. Anyone! I'd better ring home. My parents are usually in bed by now but since Jenny's out, they'll probably stay awake until she comes back from the club. But no one picks up. Even if they were asleep, they would have heard the phone by now. Something's going on. Maybe one of them has had a heart attack. Oh God. I call my aunt. If something's happened, she's bound to know.

"Hello?" Her faint voice tells me she must be unwell.

"Di? It's Melanie."

"Melanie, thank God. Your parents have been trying to get hold of you."

"What's happened? Are they OK?"

"It's your sister. She …"

"What? What's wrong with her?"

"Your mother called me to say she had been taken to hospital. She collapsed in a club, apparently. Now, what she was doing in a club at sixteen, I ask you …"

"What do you mean she collapsed?"

"Apparently she had taken drugs. Ecstasy, I think."

****

The journey to the hospital is the worst I've ever had to make. It seems the taxi driver is going as slowly as he possibly can. I keep asking him to speed up, but all he says is that "the traffic is always terrible on a Saturday night." This is the time I wish everyone had a damn mobile phone. Mine hasn't rung since I left the flat. I wonder if it's a good or a bad sign. My little sister's in hospital! She took drugs. She tried to tell me about it. That day we went shopping together; she wanted to talk and I ignored her! And if I had bothered to go to her stupid party it would probably not have happened! If she dies I'll never forgive myself. I can't believe this is happening. It can't be real; I must still be asleep, sitting on the sofa in front of the television; yes, that's right. It's that damn wine, giving me nightmares! I pinch myself but nothing happens. I pinch again, harder and harder, until the skin turns red and starts to bleed. But I'm still in the cab. I'm still in that damn fucking cab!

"Excuse me, lady, are you alright?" The driver asks, his big eyes staring at me through his mirror.

"How long left until we get there?"

"I'd say maybe twenty minutes, love. All these people coming back from the pub, makes the roads busy!"

"Are you sure you're taking the quickest ways?"

"Course I am! I'm not one of those bloody minicabs! Nightmare, they are. They're a shame to our business, I tell you! And they're all foreigners, can't hold a bloody conversation with them!" And he doesn't see the irony. "So what you're going to the hospital for, love?"

"Look, can we just drive? I'm sorry but I'm really not in the mood." He mumbles something and finally cuts his microphone off. I should have got on the tube. Why didn't I think about that? And that would have cost me about a hundred times less.

When we finally arrive, I jump out of the cab and run to the reception area. I've never been in a hospital before. There are people everywhere, standing, sitting, lying on the chairs. Thankfully I don't have to queue long to speak to the receptionist.

"My sister was taken here about two hours ago."

"Melanie?" I turn around to see my mother and father running towards me. Their eyes are red and swollen, and they're both shaking. "You've made it at last!"

"What happened? Is she OK?" My mother bursts into tears.

"Drugs! She took drugs! My little baby! She's only sixteen, Melanie! How could she?"

"She's stable", my father finally says. "Thankfully, she threw up just before collapsing. She will be OK. Did she ever mention anything to you? Do you know how long this has been going on? Melanie?"

"No. But … But I'm sure it was just a one off. She's not that kind of girl." But as I say this I realise that I don't actually know. Maybe it wasn't the first time. I just assumed. If I had spoken to her when she wanted to …

"Why weren't you there?" My mother says between two sobs.

"I ..."

"And why didn't you pick up your phone? What's the point of having a mobile if you don't pick it up?"

"Eunice, calm down. It's not her fault. Come on, we should all sit down and wait for the doctor." The last thing I need is a sermon. What is she trying to do? Does she think I don't care or something?

"You should have been there," she continues, staring at me with anger. "She invited you! What were you doing that was so important?"

"Eunice."

"Go on! Tell me. What was more important than to spend time with your family?" If I open my mouth now I'm going to explode. I try really hard not to let anything out. I bite my lips and look at the television screen to distract myself. A homeless man is lying on the chairs in front of me, snoring, and from time to time opening his eyes to turn sides. Another one is standing by the reception desk, talking loudly and making wide gestures, occasionally hitting the people who walk past. My father puts a hand on my leg and forces a smile. I smile back, conscious that my mother is behind him, looking at me with pain and anger in eyes. Yes, it is my fault. But do I deserve such hatred? I didn't mean for her to be here. How does she think I feel? I haven't seen her that angry since I broke her favourite vase. She nearly killed me. For a vase! If Jenny dies, she'll blame me forever. She'll probably accuse me of giving her the damn drugs!

After the doctor came to tell us that Jenny wouldn't suffer from any long term damage, I went back home. My parents stayed, and they will have probably spent the whole night there, but I couldn't face another minute in that place. I couldn't face my mother's abuse, and even less seeing Jenny. I don't know what I would have done if she had died. I spend the next day walking around aimlessly in the streets, trying to get my head cleared of all the mess. I get on a train, and eventually, without really knowing why, I end up on Naomi's doorstep. The chances of her being in are always minimal these days, but to my surprise she opens the door.

"Mel! What ... what a surprise."

"Can I come in?"

"Sure. I was just about to take a break."

"From what?"

"From my revision! My oral is next week, remember? I told you I was taking summer classes."

"Ah, yes. Sorry."

"So, what brings you here?"

"I ... I was just in the area; I thought I'd say hi."

"What were you doing around here? You always say you hate this part of London." It's a lie. I only say that because I'm jealous that she lives in Greenwich and I live in scruffy land. Her parents pay for the rent, which is cheaper than mine.

"I know. I was walking and I ended up here."

"You walked from Turnpike Lane?"

"I'm not that mad. I got the train." I say impatiently.

"Right. Do you … want something to drink?"

"No, thanks."

"So … what did you get up to last night?"

"I had to go to hospital."

"Why? What happened? Are you alright?"

"It wasn't me. It was Jenny. She'd taken drugs."

"Oh my God. Jenny? But … what is she, sixteen?"

"Yeah."

"That's so sad … is she OK?"

"She'll be fine. I think she just needs to stay in hospital for a couple of nights, but she's out of danger."

"Wasn't yesterday her birthday party?"

"Yes."

"That's horrible. Just horrible. Kids, these days. How long had she been taking drugs for?"

"I don't know."

"I guess not. It's not the kind of things you talk to your family about, really."

"She told me."

"What?"

"When we went shopping. She tried to talk to me about it. I ignored her." My whole body's shaking. I can see without looking at her that she's gradually getting more and more shocked.

"I don't understand. Why would you do that?"

"I don't know. I didn't think."

"You didn't think? Your own sister tells you she takes drugs and you ignore her?"

"She didn't say she took drugs."

"But she tried to. I mean, you've just said …"

"I … I …" I'm out of words. My head's such a mess. I don't even know why I told her.

"I don't believe you! Actually, no, it doesn't surprise me. You're so self-centred! You're so obsessed with yourself that you never listen to anyone else's problems!"

"That's bullshit! I really don't need this right now." I get up and head for the door.

"See? That's what I mean! You run away from everything."

"That's not true."

"Oh really? So you think your attitude is normal, do you?"

"What is that even supposed to mean?"

"You don't think you have any issues?"

"I don't know what you're talking about!"

"Every time I try to talk to you about your weight, or your alcohol abuse, or anything else that worries me, you run away. When I try to tell you about my own problems, you're not interested. And when I finally meet someone who makes me happy, you try to ruin it!"

"I didn't try to ruin anything!"

"What about the restaurant? You nearly scared him off!"

"It's not my fault if we didn't get on!"

"But you don't get on with anyone! You never give anyone a chance! And someone died because you wouldn't help them!" I can't believe she brought that up.

She's the one who told me to forget about it at the time. She's the one who made it seem half as important as her stupid date!

"You told me it wasn't my fault."

"Because you were upset and I was trying to make you feel better! But to be honest, if you had opened your door, she'd probably still be alive!"

"Shut up."

"Why, does the truth hurt?"

"Shut the fuck up!" As she stands in front of me, I can barely control myself. I want to hit her. I want to beat her down and kick the shit out of her. My heart is beating so fast I can hardly breathe.

"You need to sort yourself out, Melanie. Because if you don't, no one else will do it for you, and more people will get hurt." I can't stay here and let her try to bring me down. Stupid cow! She deserves that boring bastard. And I don't need to waste anymore of my time with such a prat. So I go, despite an unbearable urge to hurt her. I stop at the nearest off licence and buy a couple of ciders. After a few sips, I feel much better. When I think of how mad she looked, it's almost funny. As for me, from now on I'm going to concentrate on the only person who's worth my time and energy; he's coming over soon and I can hardly contain my excitement. I stop in a couple of shops and try things on, which I hadn't done for as long as I can remember. And I actually find clothes to buy! Then, I go to a coffee shop and sit at a table, half reading the magazine I bought and half looking at the people around me. And I enjoy it. The thought of having a purpose, a goal in my life, or at least for the next two weeks, lifts me up in the most satisfying way … Even if I might just have lost the one person I thought was a friend.

The next few days, my mood doesn't change much. At work, people tell me I look good and happy! I haven't told anyone what's going on of course; they'd only laugh! Meeting someone on the Internet! But you read stories about it all the time these days; people fall in love online, marry, have children. Not that I'm thinking of that obviously! I don't even know what Simon looks like, let alone our children! I wonder where we'd get married. I don't want anything big and I don't think he would either. There wouldn't be many people to invite anyway! And there wouldn't be a photographer. Or maybe one that would just take pictures of him! I'd love to have pictures of him. I'm sure he's handsome. He's so bright, he has to be handsome. And he would be, in his white tuxedo! It would have to be white. And I'd have to wear a black dress. It would be a great wedding. And I would invite Naomi, just to make her jealous because our wedding would be far better than hers! But I won't mention any of this on our first date, obviously. He'd think I'm mad! I wonder how he'll propose. Maybe he'll take me to a very expensive restaurant, order some champagne and in front of all the other dinners he'll get on his knees and reveal before me the biggest, most colourful and bright stone. And when I say yes, everyone will cheer us! I can't wait. And I'll move to the States! Yes! He'll find me a great job in his company, maybe I'll be able to do it from home, and I'll have lots of friends, because the people there are so nice! Oh God, I'm so excited.

I don't hear from him until two days before we're supposed to meet, but I know how busy he is so it doesn't bother me. I was hoping to see him a bit earlier than originally planned, but it doesn't matter if we're going to spend the rest of our lives together. We arrange to meet at Café Med in Notting Hill, which is quite far away from me but apparently close to his hotel. I spend the evening before trying on different outfits, applying makeup and doing my hair; and I actually enjoy it! I make a list of what I've decided to wear (in case I forget!) and the things I should/should not talk to him about. But we've already said so much online, I struggle to find anything new! I'm so nervous and overjoyed that I don't get any sleep and for fear of being late, I arrive an hour early. So I sit in a café not far from the restaurant, not daring to look up too much in case he's around; I don't want him to think I'm a sad cow with nothing to do other than waiting around for him! I try to read the paper I got (Financial Times – since he's a business man, I figured it'd look good if I met him with it in my hand), but I can't concentrate at all. The hour seems like a day. I'm nervous of course, but mostly impatient.

I just want this day to end, so we can move on to the next date when it will be far less awkward and scary. But maybe once we're face to face, it won't be awkward at all! Maybe we'll click instantly. There's no reason why we wouldn't, we already know each other so well. I don't know whether to arrive early or late; if I'm late he might think I'm rude, and if I'm early, that I'm desperate. So at 12:59pm, I leave the café and aim for the restaurant.

I don't know who to look for; all he said was that he'd be waiting at a table outside; it would have been easier to know what he looked like, or what he was wearing, but since he didn't say, I didn't dare to ask.

Which now seems very silly; what if there are ten different men sitting alone? From the distance, the tables all seem to be occupied; so instead of wandering around like an idiot in search of a lone man, I decide to ring him.

"I'm here!" he says, as a man gets up and starts looking around. Then he sees me, and waves. This is it. There's no turning back now. I try to smile as I get closer to him, and he smiles back; he seems pleased to see me. He's not exactly like I had imagined him; his hair is mousy brown, his eyes are somewhere between green and grey, and he's a bit shorter than me. He's wearing a dark blue suit and a black tie, and despite the fact that he has a couple of gold rings on his right hand and his hair seems overly gelled, he's still fairly attractive.

"Hello, Melanie! It's so nice to meet you at last", he shouts, grabbing my hand to shake it.

"You too!" I reply in a shaky voice.

"Please, take a seat. What would you like to drink?" All I can see on the table is a glass of water.

"I'll ... I'll have some water, please." If I order anything else he'll probably think I'm an alcoholic. Part of me had expected to start the lunch with champagne.

"Excuse me, waiter, can I get a glass of water for the lady?" he shouts at the nearest employee, who seems fairly annoyed by his interjection. I can see half the people at the tables around us giving us funny looks.

"So ... How has your week been so far?" I ask, trying to lighten the atmosphere.

"Pretty cool! I'm just about to close a great deal. I haven't seen much of the scenery of course, I've been way too busy."

"Of course!" I repeat, as though I knew exactly what it was like to be a businessman. "Are you planning to do any sight-seeing?"

"I don't know really! It all kind of seems a bit dull here."

I don't particularly like London, but I wouldn't say it was dull; and I certainly wouldn't say New York was dull to a New Yorker if I'd only been in their town five minutes.

"There are some really nice places to see, actually. It depends where you go …"

"Yeah, no doubt. Didn't I order some water?" he asks, looking around.

"I'm sure it will arrive soon. Don't … don't worry about it." But as soon as he sees a waiter, he calls him.

"Excuse me? I ordered some water."

"Yes, sir," he replies politely, and after putting down on the table the three plates he was carrying, disappears back inside.

"So, let's have a peek at that menu, shall we? Will you have a starter?"

"Err … No, I think I'll just have a salad."

"A salad? Like, lettuce and stuff?" He grabs a piece of bread, and sinks half of it in his mouth, chewing loudly.

"Well … Yes, that kind of thing." He raises his eyebrows, in a "how weird and boring" way.

"You don't mind if I get something a little bit more substantial, do you?" he says with what sounds like a snore.

"No, of course." Thankfully, the waiter arrives shortly after with my water; I was getting worried Simon might start shouting at somebody else soon.

"I'll have the smoked salmon for starter, and the steak and fries for main, with extra fries. I know you guys aren't too generous with the portions!" He laughs, pointing at the table in front of us. "What are you having, Melanie?" I hadn't actually thought about it yet, so I quickly scan the salads.

"I … I'll have the Caesar salad, please, with no sauce."

"No sauce? Are you on a diet or something?" I feel myself blush.

"No, I just … don't like sauce."

"Fair enough!" he says with another snore. "Can we make it quite quick please, I only have about an hour", he says to the waiter whilst handing him the menus back.

"We're very busy as you can see sir, but we'll do our best." He only has an hour. He never mentioned that on the phone.

"So … what have you got planned this afternoon?" I ask, trying not to sound disappointed.

"I've got a couple of meetings; you know what it's like, places to be, people to see."

"Sure. They don't give you much free time, do they?"

"They don't, but I don't mind. More work means more money."

"Right." So money's more important than spending time with me, I want to say. It doesn't matter that I've been waiting months for this day. It doesn't matter that I spent the whole evening preparing for it. He wants to make money. Now I understand why he doesn't have friends. What I don't understand is that online, he was a completely different person. Kind, funny, intelligent. I am having lunch with a rude, annoying and inconsiderate pig.

"So, how's your sister doing?" He asks casually, as if he were talking about the weather.

"She's better. Much better." Somehow I don't feel like giving him too much detail; I'm scared he might say something offensive.

"That's good." I was expecting a bit more support, somehow; but I'm starting to feel I might be wasting my time. I have a sudden urge to get up and leave; but then I remember what Naomi said about running away from my problems. I have to prove her wrong.

"It's funny; when we were online you seemed different."

"In what way?" he says his mouth full of bread.

"I just never realised you were so focused on money."

"I guess I don't consider the web as something real; I mean, don't get me wrong, there are a lot of real things happening on the net. That's how I do most of my business. It's just, talking to someone in a chat room; it's like being in a different dimension. You can be whatever you want. You can re- invent yourself completely. I love it. I'm like … this new person. Pretty much the opposite of the real me, actually! Isn't it weird?" He bursts out laughing. I struggle to find words. I struggle not to throw my water at him.

"So … the things you said on the net, they weren't real either?"

"Honey, I say a lot of things. You'd have to give me examples."

"That … won't be necessary. I'm sorry, I made a mistake." Sod what Naomi said, I can't spend another minute next to that twat. I get up and grab my bag.

"What are you doing?"

"Leaving. Now you'll have even more time for your precious money! When I think I was looking forward to meeting you, to being with you! I thought you were different. You were so different. But now you're just like the rest of them. You're just a fucking arsehole!" I can feel everyone's eyes on me, but I don't care. I can see his look of horror, of disbelief and embarrassment, and I'm pleased. I want to kill him. I want him to feel all the pain I have inside. For cheating. For misleading me. For letting me down so badly. But I just go. Tears in my eyes, I walk away, helpless, hurt like I've never been before. It's not worth it. I've nothing left. I've lost the only thing I thought I still had. I don't have anything but myself. My body, my ugly deformed body and my soul. My bruised soul. I don't want them anymore. Twenty-one years of them is too much. I can't spend another day with them. How can it ever get better when I ache so much? Naomi was right. I do need help, and no one can help me but me. So I will do the only thing that will truly help me. End it.

Chapter 4

It's so dark. So cold. So empty. All gone. Destroyed. Ruined. I'm scared. But I refuse to spend another day, another hour, here. I walk past a million people, a million lights, all mixing into one blur. I feel empty, but yet there's so much noise in my head. I stop at the nearest off-licence, buy as much alcohol as I can afford, three boxes of Paracetamol (which I thought I might have some trouble getting, but the guy at the counter was more worried about the match he was watching on his portable TV) and razor blades. Then I sit in a park, at a quiet spot by a tree and drink, swallowing the pills slowly. I look at the people playing football, reading, kissing, and think of how lucky I am. Loss, pain, anger, diseases, poverty, rain, clouds, crowds … it's all behind me.

I remember the first time I really thought of killing myself. I was twelve. My mother had been on sleeping pills for a short while, and when she stopped, she left a full box of tablets behind. So one day, I emptied it. I must have taken about 30 pills. But what I didn't know was that they were herbal pills. Whilst swallowing, I had pictures in my head of what I had lived through so far, what I hadn't done and what I'd never get to do. The people who had hurt me and already given me a far from glorifying image of humanity; the bullying, the mocking at school after each forced trip to the hairdresser's, my mother telling me off at every opportunity, Ashley, who read out loud in class the letter I'd given him telling of my feelings for him; John, who told me I was too fat to be in his football team when we were seven. Sara, who didn't think I was pretty enough to be her friend. I waited, crying, imagining the moment my parents would find me, lying on the floor unconscious. I waited for hours, but nothing happened. I didn't even feel sick. So then I read the label more closely; and realised my stupid mistake. I laughed. I thought it was a sign that maybe I should give life a chance. Well, I did. I gave it nine more years. And what's changed? I fight the tears rolling down my face. This is no time for crying. It's probably the happiest moment of my life! I take a blade out of my bag, unwrap it, and put it on my wrist. Slowly, I run it up and down, gently at first, and look at the tiny drops of blood. Then I press harder and harder, my skin opening up. I swallow more pills, drink more wine and watch my arm turning red. After a while, a couple of hours maybe, I'm starting to feel sleepy. I lean against the tree and close my eyes. It's happening.

"Excuse me, Madam, have you got the time?" A man is standing in front of me and even though my vision is blurry I can tell by the look on his face that he probably knows what I'm doing. He bends down, staring at my arms, then at the empty bottles. I don't know why, but I burst out laughing.

"What's happened here? Are you OK?"

"I'm great, thanks! Want to join my party?" I say giggling. I can't help it, it's just too funny.

"Can I look at your arms?" I'd run if my legs allowed me to, but I can't even move my fingers. He grabs my arm and makes a noise close to a sigh, or disgust. I can't really tell.

"Just wait here for a second." He gets up, moves a couple of metres away and starts talking on his phone. Whilst he's not looking I down a couple more pills.

"An ambulance is on its way. I'll wait with you."

"An ambulance? What are you talking about? I don't need an ambulance!"

"Have you taken any of these?" He asks, holding the box of pills.

"Just … a couple. I … had a head … ache."

"It's almost empty. Were you trying to kill yourself?"

"No, of course not! Who … do you think I am? I told you, I … had a headache!"

"What's happened to your arms then? Is that some new trend I don't know about?"

"I … I tried to climb up that tree and I scratched them!" I can't stop laughing. But he doesn't seem remotely amused. I wish he'd sod off!

"How many pills have you taken? Can you remember?"

"You've got the box, sir, I'm sure you can count, can't you?" He's really starting to annoy me. Not only do people screw up your life but they won't even let you die in peace!

"There they are." Who? What? I feel dizzy. My head is spinning badly. What's going on? I'm confused. Two figures appear out of nowhere in front of me, giving me a fright.

"Hi Madam, can you try to get up?"

"Why …? No … I … I can't move."

The next few hours come in a string of flashes. An ambulance. A hospital bed. A nurse telling me off for throwing up. A needle in my arm. People shouting. Someone asking me if I can go and sit in the waiting room because they need my bed. Why do I need to stay here anyway? I may as well go home. I don't like being told off. Especially by a damn nurse. I mean, she's paid to look after sick people, not to have a go at them!

"Excuse me, please take a seat, someone will be with you soon." The bitch nurse grabs my arm as I'm about to walk out.

"But why? I've been here hours. What else are you planning to do to me?"

"Someone will come to talk to you soon." She makes me sit down, and then says something to the security guard, about me, no doubt, as he gives me a suspicious look. I wonder what he'd do if I tried to go again. Attack me, probably. It's freezing in here; there's hardly anyone around. It reminds me of Jenny. How worried my parents were. I wonder if they'd feel the same now. Mother would probably have a go at me for being an attention seeker.

About three hours later, when I'm starting to think and see more clearly, I'm taken into a small blue room by a tall, skinny man with dreadlocks and a shorter, bald one. Neither of them looks much older than me.

"Melanie, is that right?" Asks the dreadlocked guy.

"Yes."

"I'm James, psychiatric nurse, and this is doctor Schoenberg." The doctor in question gives me a half-hearted smile.

"So ... Can you tell us what happened tonight?" What am I supposed to say to that? They're obviously expecting something in the line of: "I tried to kill myself"; why do they bother asking since they already know the answer?

"I fancied a trip to the hospital." For a moment they sit silently.

"And why is that? A hospital isn't the nicest place to be in", the doctor finally says.

"I was bored."

"Did you harm yourself tonight?"

"I suppose so."

"Had you done anything like this before?" This is so uncomfortable. I feel like I'm a schoolgirl getting told off.

"I'm sorry but I'd like to go home. You're wasting your time with me." As I get up, the dreadlocked guy does the same.

"Please, sit down. We just want to help you."

"Then let me go!"

"What would you do if we did let you go?"

"I'd go home to bed."

"Do you live with anyone?"

"No." I realise straight away that I should have said yes.

"So you would be alone."

"No. I'd ... I'd invite a friend over. I have a lot of friends."

"At this time? Are you sure someone could come over?" I hadn't noticed the clock above the door. It's a quarter to two.

"Yes."

"How have you been feeling recently? Has anything happened in your life that might have made you want to kill yourself?"

"No. It was just the alcohol. Everything's … great."

"What about your past? Your childhood? Your teens?"

"Look, I've had a normal life. Everyone has problems. I'm fine. I'm just very tired now."

"Melanie, for your own safety I don't think letting you go would be a good idea." What is he talking about? What does he want to do with me?

"I told you, I'll be fine, I just want to go to bed now!"

"Would you mind just waiting a couple of minutes, we have to discuss the situation with our team. We will be back shortly."

"What situation? What team?"

"It's just standard procedure. Can I get you anything? Coffee? Water?"

"You could call me a cab!"

"Please, bear with us." They get up and go, leaving the door wide open. There's a board in the hall in front of me and my name is on it, followed by the letters "NTL". It takes me a while to figure out what it means: "Not To Leave". I'm about to run out when I notice someone standing by the door. A security guard. I have my own security guard!

****

An hour. It's been a whole hour since they left. I'm now almost completely sober and as each minute that passes is making me less and less drunk, the more the whole thing is starting to be unbearable. Is this a test to see how long it's going to take me before I lose my mind completely? "They won't be long", the security guard keeps saying. Or maybe they were waiting for me to sober up, so they can send me home knowing I'm in the right state of mind! Yes, that would make sense. I'm annoyed that they didn't say so to begin with, but now at least I have hope. Maybe a coffee would speed up the process.

"Excuse me? Can I get a coffee, please?" I ask the security guy in my most polite voice. Although what I'm dying to say is "Is this what you get paid for? Guarding doors?"

"I'll get it. What would you like?"

"Err ..." I wasn't expecting that answer. "Can't I just go and buy it myself? I mean, the machine's just there!" I say pointing at the vending machine about five metres away.

"Sorry, but you can't leave the room."

"What if I need the toilet?"

"Then I'd have to come with you."

"This is a fucking joke, right?"

"What would you like to drink?" he repeats. I realise insulting or punching him probably won't help, so I just ask for a black coffee. Ironically, as I sit down the doctor comes back, with a woman I haven't met yet.

"Sorry to have kept you waiting. This is Doctor Morris; she works at the St Mary's Hospital."

"Hi, Melanie."

"Hi. I'm feeling much better now", I say as cheerfully and apologetically as I can. "I've sobered up. I'm really sorry about what happened tonight."

"There's nothing to be sorry about, Melanie. I am here because I have had a talk with doctor Schoenberg and even though you might be feeling better now, I don't think we should send you home just yet."

"What do you mean, just yet?"

"I would like you to come with me to St Mary's; get some rest and we could talk a bit more tomorrow."

"What do you mean? What is St Mary's? Why should I go there?"

"St Mary's is a psychiatric hospital, not far from here. They have a couple of spare beds in one of their wards, and I really feel it would be a good idea if you spent a bit of time there." I must be dreaming. No, I'm dead and I've been sent to hell.

"Sorry, but I don't need psychiatric help. I got drunk and did something stupid, it happens to a lot of people. You don't go around locking away anyone who get pissed and a bit depressed, do you?"

"But you didn't just get a bit depressed, Melanie. You tried to commit suicide."

"It is for your own good", the other Doctor finally says. "We just want you to be safe." Safe? How can I be safe if I'm sent in a place full of lunatics?

"Thanks, but I don't need your help."

"It would make things a lot easier for yourself if you agreed to come to St Mary's. Otherwise we would have to section you, and this would mean that you would have to spend much longer there."

"You mean you'd force me?"

"I am afraid so. As I said, we just cannot risk letting you go now. You said things earlier on which implied that you had a strong will to end your life."

"I said things? What things? When?"

"In the ambulance, and when the nurse was examining you. You told us many times that we should let you die and go help people who really needed us. You didn't seem to think you were one of them."

****

They put me in a taxi. They drive me to St Mary's. "Welcome to the Lordship ward. Don't worry, my dear, we'll look after you." They make me sign papers. They take me to "my" room. Give me pink and yellow flowery pyjamas, three times my size. "Get some rest, darling." Rest. That's all I've been asking for. How am I supposed to "rest" with a woman snoring, one talking to herself and another one coughing her guts out? They never said "my" room wouldn't just be mine. I pull the curtains surrounding my bed and lie on the hollow mattress. I don't have a toothbrush. Nor any clothes for tomorrow. I guess I'll probably see that woman again when I get up and she'll hopefully let me go straight away. There's a board behind the bed, with a couple of pictures on it of children. Maybe the previous occupant here had left them behind. But why would they leave pictures of their kids here? Someone's written "Help me" in red above them. I wonder if they did.

"Hello? Breakfast time." I open my eyes and see a man standing by my bed. By the time I manage to remember where I am he's already gone. I must have fallen asleep. There's a lot of noise outside; footsteps squeaking on the linoleum floor, people talking and I think I can hear cries. I wait until I'm sure all my room mates have left before opening the curtains. The walls are green and stained and there's an unmistakable smell of urine coming from the bed in front of mine.

Without intending to, I find myself facing the dusty mirror above the sink, and as much as I'm used to the obscene deformity of what is called my body, what I'm seeing beats even the lowest of the lows. I have the hair of a blind punk, my eyeliner has run all the way down to my cheeks, my lips are dry and my clothes are covered in blood and sick. I could really do with a coffee, but I don't know if there's a machine or a kitchen or if I'd have to sit with all the loonies and be force-fed. There's a hairbrush on the sink and I'm tempted to use it, but it's probably full of nits and dandruff. I comb my hair with my fingers, splash water on my face and try to rub off as many of the stains on my clothes as I can. Most of these people would probably not be able to tell the difference between a human being and a vegetable, but I need to look presentable for the doctor. Then, feeling deeply apprehensive, I come out. I walk down a long corridor, towards what looks like an office. I pass a large room furnished with brown leather-like sofas and a wide-screen TV, but I don't see anyone. They're probably all eating; this place must be full of bulimics. I knock on the office door; a short and large black woman opens it, and welcomes me with a grimace.

"You're the new girl?"

"Y ... Yes. I was wondering if I could see the doctor."

"The doctor doesn't come until this afternoon."

"Melanie, is it? A man behind her gets up and shakes my hand. "I'm Ali, the ward manager. Have you had breakfast?"

"No, I'm not hungry; what time is the doctor coming?"

"This afternoon", the large woman says again. I was hoping Ali would give me a better answer.

"Do you know what time?"

"No, dear. Why don't you sit in the lounge and watch some TV?" And risk meeting the psychos?

"Actually, I'd like to have a shower, please." I am taken to what could be easily mistaken for a camping or swimming pool cabin. "Have you got a towel and some shower gel? And some shampoo and conditioner as well, please?" She looks at me as though I'd asked her for a box of chocolates.

"I'll see." She comes back ten minutes later with a cloth-sized towel and some soap. "It works for your hair too." But I give up trying to wash it as it takes me half an hour to rinse off all the soap on my body, the shower head being stuck to the wall without a cable, and the water coming out in drips. As the door lock is broken, I spend the whole time worrying that someone might come in, either to shower or to assault me. I wonder what that woman would have said if I'd asked her for clean clothes. I put on my socks and underwear inside out; thankfully my t-shirt is stain-free as I wore a cardigan on top of it, so I decide to discard the latter, even if that means freezing to death … not such a bad idea, come to think of it. I go back to the office, looking down and walking fast to make sure no one tries to talk to me; I ask for a deodorant and hairbrush. "We don't have any. Ask your room mates." Yes, of course. I'd rather stink than share anything with these freaks.

"I need to see the doctor!" Someone shouts behind me. I turn around in surprise, and am faced with the tiniest, skinniest woman I've ever seen. Her black hair is messier than mine and her eyes are red and swollen. "I need to see the doctor!" She repeats more loudly.

"The doctor's not here. He's coming this afternoon."

"But I need to see him now! I've hurt my leg!"

"What's wrong with it?" The large woman says reluctantly, not moving from her chair.

"I don't know, do I? Or I wouldn't want a doctor to look at it!" Ali finally comes out of the office.

"Have you been drinking, Jean?"

"Just look at my leg!" She walks a couple of steps backwards, defensively. She looks frightened, as if she were expecting him to hit her.

"You know the rules, Jean. You're not allowed to drink on the grounds!"

"I didn't drink on the grounds, I was outside! And I only had one! At least give me some pain killers if I can't see the doctor!"

"We can't give you anything whilst you're under the influence of alcohol. You know that." As her eyes suddenly meet mine, I quickly look down and aim back to my room. I find a large, grey-haired woman in a green, traditional-looking dress, standing by my bed.

"Hello! You new?"

"Yes." She claps her hands and starts dancing and singing in what sounds like Greek or Turkish. Maybe I should go look for a vending machine. I check my purse for coins – it's empty. How can that be? I'm sure I had money in it yesterday. I must have had, otherwise how would I have paid for the drinks and pills? I bet someone stole from me! But I kept my bag with me everywhere. Maybe they took the money whilst I was asleep. I should have known. I should have hidden my purse in the bed. I don't think there was much in it though, a few pounds maybe. How low of them! Thankfully, they didn't take my cards. So now I need a cash machine on top of everything. In the hall I spot a woman wearing a badge, another nurse probably, so I ask her where the nearest ATM is.

"There aren't any", she says dryly.

"Surely there are outside?"

"You can't go outside."

"I can't go outside?" I repeat, baffled.

"No."

"But I need money!"

"What for?"

"Coffee."

"You don't need to pay for coffee. Didn't you get some at breakfast?"

"No, I didn't go for breakfast." She frowns.

"Well, you should have. There is a tea break in an hour. You can have coffee then." But I need coffee now!

"I want to see a fucking doctor!" I can hear the skinny drunk woman scream. She's still standing outside the office.

"I told you the doctor isn't coming until this afternoon! You need to sober up, drink some water and go watch TV or something!" The large nurse says quite aggressively.

"Don't you tell me what to do! You wouldn't treat me like that if I was black, would you? You guys are all racist! You can't go around treating white people like shit, you know? If you don't like us then go back to your own country!"

"That's enough now, go back to your room!" Two men come out of the office and grab her arms.

"No! Don't touch me!" she screams even more loudly than before. But the men pull her forward and she falls over.

"My leg! You bastards! You've hurt my leg!" Jean is now lying on the floor, holding her leg with both hands. She seems in pain.

"Come on, get up. I haven't got all day", one of the men says, bending down.

"You bastards!" Jean repeats. "You racist bastards! I won't move until you've called the doctor! You won't get away with this!"

"Call security", Ali says to the large woman. She runs into her office. A minute later, two security guards appear. They try to grab hold of Jean, but she struggles violently, pushing them away a few times before they manage to immobilise her. She still tries to resist, screaming and crying hysterically, as if she thought they were going to kill her. She's taken into what I guess is her room, followed by a couple of nurses, one of them holding a syringe. They close the door behind them, leaving the whole place in a deep and heavy silence.

"You racist bastards!" an old woman with giant glasses shouts from the TV room. I feel numb. I can't move. I've never seen anything like this before. She seemed so distressed, so scared. I wonder if they were really trying to help her and she didn't realise because she was drunk, or if they deliberately hurt her. Are they used to this kind of behaviour and that's why they dealt with it so coldly? Or has this just never happened before and they didn't know how to handle it? It's quite shocking, really, whatever their excuse. A blonde girl is walking up and down the corridors, talking to herself vacantly. As she goes past me, she stops and smiles. I don't know why, but I smile back. I wait for her to say something, but she doesn't. She looks deep into my eyes and starts walking again.

"Tea time!" the nurse with the syringe says loudly. People come out of their rooms and follow her into the lounge. They all stand behind her and wait for her to unlock a door, which I guess leads to the kitchen or a tea area. I hesitate for a moment, and then decide to join them. I desperately need caffeine. I don't have to talk to anyone; I'll just get my drink and mind my own business. There's about ten of us; the blonde girl, the woman with giant glasses, the Turkish one, plus others that I haven't seen before. We walk down some stairs, towards what looks like a school canteen. We join a queue of about fifteen more people, both men and women. I wonder where they came from. There's bread, white and brown, jam, butter, and thankfully, a coffee machine; with a large choice of coffees, teas and hot chocolate. I take a cup and sit at an empty table. I don't look up, although part of me is dying to.

"Excuse me, can I sit here?" A young, pretty girl dressed in a black fishnet top and short skirt is standing in front of me, holding a tray. She smiles shyly.

"Err … Sure."

"Are you the new girl in Lordship?"

"Yeah."

"Hi. I'm Sam." She gives me her hand to shake.

"Melanie."

"Nice to meet you, Melanie. Can I ask what brought you here?" I'm embarrassed. I contemplate making up a story, but by the time I find one that would be credible enough she'd probably have given up listening.

"I ... I took some pills."

"Attempted suicide?" The words echo in my head like a song out of tune.

"Yes."

"Same here. Is it your first time in a place like this?"

"Yes. But I'm only here for today. I'm waiting for the doctor to come and then I'll be off."

"So soon? They told me they'd keep me a couple of days and I've been here for two months." Huh.

"Hello!"

"Hi, Paul. This is Melanie, she's new."

"Hi, Melanie" A tall, slim man wearing clothes that make him look about fifty, sits next to Sam.

"Welcome to the mad house. What are you here for?"

"Same as me", Sam says, as though she'd sensed I didn't want to repeat myself.

"How old are you?"

"Twenty-one."

"I'm twenty. Sam's seventeen." Seventeen. She's in a mental institution at seventeen. And I thought I had it bad.

"How long have you been here for?" I find myself asking Paul.

"A month and a half."

"Paul's manic depressive" Sam adds.

"And Sam's just depressive", Paul says, smiling. I want to ask him about his mania, but I fear the answer. I'm not used to talking about that kind of thing.

"So there are men as well here? I hadn't noticed any until now."

"We're in different wards. There are two for women and two for men. We meet on tea and food breaks and during activities. Were you hoping for a women-only environment?" He asks, still smiling.

"Oh, no", I say defensively, "I just didn't realise there was more than one ward."

"Yeah. There's lots of us loonies around. Have to keep us in separate cages", he adds laughing. Surprisingly, I don't feel as tense as I did an hour ago. We talk about what we did before coming here, what the people are like ("Mad, obviously, but harmless. You should be more scared of the staff. They're all wankers.") Then we're asked to go back upstairs. I sit in the lounge with Sam and watch some TV, keeping an eye on the clock. I wonder what time they meant by "this afternoon". One o'clock? Two? Surely no later than that. The lunch break comes fairly quickly; the food is surprisingly tasty. Of course I don't have much of it (a bit of salad, rice and vegetables – no dessert). I'm welcomed by a couple more people, one of them called Jeff, who claims to be "a Catholic, a Jew, a Muslim and a Pagan. I'm not gay, but if you are it doesn't matter." ("No, I'm not, but thanks") and another called Mourad, who promises me £ 10,000 when he comes out, what he will get after divorcing his wife – who I am told by Paul died two years ago. After lunch I go see the nurses.

"The doctor came. There was a situation with one of the patients, as you probably noticed. He left ten minutes ago. But you will see him tomorrow."

"What? What do you mean he came? You told me he would see me this afternoon! I've been waiting all day to see him! I can't wait until tomorrow; I'm supposed to leave today!" I'm struggling to speak.

"Who said that?"

"The doctor I saw yesterday. She said I'd get some rest here and see someone this morning!"

"But she didn't mean you would leave today, dear. We can't just let you go after one night." I can't believe this. I just can't.

"But … but … I can't stay here! I have things to do; I have to go to work tomorrow!"

"Well then you shouldn't have come here in the first place, should you? You should have thought of the implications."

"But I didn't want to come here! I was forced!"

"And for good reasons. I'm sorry you couldn't see the doctor today, but he wouldn't have let you go anyway."

"How the fuck do you know that?"

"You watch your language." Suddenly what happened to Jean comes back to me in a flash.

"But you don't know that! Maybe he would have seen that I'm perfectly normal and would have sent me home!"

"Darling, you tried to kill yourself. You don't just get better overnight."

"But … I haven't got any clothes … I … haven't got a toothbrush … I haven't got anything!"

"You can ask someone to bring your things over." Who the hell would I call and tell I'm in a fucking mental hospital? "I'm sorry. I have to answer that." She picks up the phone which I hadn't heard ringing and answers it with a long sigh, as if she was relieved not to have to talk to me anymore. I bet she's made the call up so I'd leave her alone. I feel so stupid. So scared. I don't belong here! How long are they planning to keep me for? What the hell am I going to do about my clothes? I need Naomi. But she hates me now. And what would she think of this? And what about work? I'm supposed to be there tomorrow. This is so unfair. I run to my room, tears rolling down my eyes, and let myself fall on the bed. I cry so much I feel sick.

"Are you OK?" The blonde girl from the corridor is standing by the door, playing with her hands nervously as if she was scared I might jump on her.

"Yeah, I'm great!" I was hoping my rudeness would make her go away, but a second later she's sitting on my bed.

"Don't worry, you'll be OK. Why are you sad?" Why am I sad? Because my life is shit? Would I be here if I weren't sad?

"They won't let me go", I say dryly.

"I'm sorry. How long do they want to keep you for?"

"I don't know. I was supposed to see a doctor today but I was told I'm going to have to wait until tomorrow because he's too busy."

"Tomorrow's not very long. Maybe they will let you go after you've seen him."

"I doubt it. But I can't stay here; I haven't got any clothes, or anything, not even a fucking toothbrush!"

"You can ask someone to bring you some stuff?"

"No! No one knows I'm here." I wish she'd leave me alone.

"There's a washing machine, so you can clean your clothes. And ask them for a toothbrush, I'm sure they have spare ones."

"Thanks." But it's not just that, is it? I have nothing. If anyone knew I was here they'd freak out. Why didn't they let me die? They're punishing me. What does it matter to them whether I'm alive or not?

"Why are you here? You don't have to tell me if you don't want to." People have asked me so many times today, I don't even care about telling them anymore.

"Attempted suicide. You?" I'm half expecting her to say something like "I'm a compulsive walker." But her expression suddenly changes; she looks nervous, or angry, I can't tell.

"I hear voices. Sometimes." I never imagined I'd be one day face to face with someone like her. I thought these things only happened on TV.

"What … kind of voices?"

"I don't know." I wonder if I've upset her. Or maybe she's hearing those voices right now.

"What do they say?"

"I … don't know. It's hard to explain."

"Have you always been like this?"

"No. It only started last April."

"Really? That's only a few months ago."

"Only?" She says sarcastically, her hand running in her hair nervously.

"How did it start?" Maybe I should leave her alone, but I can't help wanting to know more.

"I don't know. It just … did."

"Have you been here since April then?"

"No, I've only been here for a few weeks."

"What were you doing before?"

"I was a PA in an insurance company." She's looking around in agitation.

"Is the food nice here?" I ask, trying to change the subject. "Lunch was alright, wasn't it?" Her face lights up again.

"Yes. It usually is. There's always nice dessert."

"Oh, I don't eat dessert, I'm too fat. As long as there are vegetables I'm happy!" She gives me a horrified look.

"But … you're not fat at all!"

"Oh, I am. I have the largest waist in the universe. You could land a plane on it!" She giggles. "I don't know your name, by the way? I'm Melanie."

"Lea."

"That's a nice name." She smiles again. The door opens and the Turkish woman walks in, singing to herself.

"I'm going for a smoke", Lea says as she gets up. "I'll see you later."

"She's mad!" The Turkish woman says as Lea leaves.

"No, shit", I laugh. But don't think she gets my sarcasm.

"Yes, she is! She hears voices and all!"

"And you don't think you're mad?" She gives me the coldest look and for a moment I think she might lynch me. But she just turns around and resumes her singing. I pull the curtains around my bed and take my phone out of my bag to ring work. I don't know what to say to them. Maybe I shouldn't bother. If I didn't show up they might call my parents as I put their names down as contacts in case of emergency; then my parents would ring Naomi and everyone would be worried sick. They'd think, "I hope she's OK. I was horrible to her; I love her, really!" But then I'd get hassle from them all instead of just work. I stare at the blank screen on my phone; it looks like it's out of battery. Just what I need. I don't bother asking the Turkish woman for a charger, as I doubt she's even got a toothbrush; I go straight to the nurses' office.

"We don't give out cables."

"I'm not asking for a cable, I'm asking for a phone charger."

"Phone chargers have cables."

"But … what's wrong with cables?"

"You could use it to strangle yourself." So that explains the showerhead. This is surreal.

"But I need to use my phone! I won't kill myself with it; I just want to charge it!"

"You can use the payphone in the hall."

"But I don't have any money and you won't let me go out and get some!" These people are really starting to get on my nerves. I don't even think any of them can speak proper English.

"You can charge your phone here", Ali says finally.

"Err … I don't really want to leave my phone here."

"Why not? Nothing's going to happen to it", the nurse replies, clearly offended.

"You can use this one", Ali adds, pointing at a phone on the nurse's desk. "Are you ringing your family?"

"No. Work. To say that I'm not coming in tomorrow. How long am I likely to stay here? I need to tell them." I dread the answer.

"It depends on you, really. We tend not to keep anyone for less than five days." Five days here? Five days of wearing the same clothes and not washing my hair? Five days of sleeping in the same room as those pigs?

"Can I change rooms, please?" I ask the nurse, trembling, after telling work I've twisted my ankle. "Do you have any individual ones?" She gives me the most evil look, and then laughs.

"This is the NHS, love, not a five-star hotel!"

"Does that mean no then?"

"Don't worry, you'll get used to your roommates", Ali says with fake compassion. "It'll take time, but you'll be OK." I want to hit him. How dare he patronise me? And how dare she laugh at me? Those people are evil! How is anyone supposed to get better in here? This is worse than a prison!

****

Am I really mad? Have I spent my whole life ignoring the possibility that there might actually be something wrong with me? Is that why I've never had friends? Because I'm different? Is that why my parents have always treated me differently from Jenny? I was born wrong and everyone but me knew it. They want to keep me here until Thursday.

"Have you ever taken any anti-depressants?" the doctor asked when I finally got to see him.

92

"No."

"Have you ever had counselling?"

"No." He made me talk about my childhood, my teens, did I get on with my parents, have I got friends to talk to, what would be the first thing I'd do when discharged. I wanted to reply "I'll try harder", but I just said "have a bath and put some new clothes on." At the end he told me he'd refer me to a therapist when I come out. I didn't argue; as long as I can go home I don't care what he plans to do with me.

"I've got at least another month", Sam tells me at lunch, a sad look on her face.

"What are you going to do when you come out?"

"I don't know. I wanted to go to college but I don't think I could handle it. I'm contemplating doing glamour modelling or something." I nearly choke.

"What? But you're only seventeen!"

"I know, but I can easily pass for twenty-three."

"That's not what I meant. You've got your whole life in front of you. Why would you want to lower yourself to that?"

"It's great money. I mean, we're talking hundreds just for one photo shoot. Don't look so disgusted! It's only pictures."

"So you don't mind the thought of old men wanking over them?"

"It's not as bad as you think. It's not like being a prostitute or anything."

"What's the difference?" From the look on her face, I don't think she knows the answer.

"See this guy with the beard over there? He sent me this text." She hands me her phone. "I can't stop thinking about you. Crazy, don't you think?"

"He wrote that? That's disgusting. He must be at least fifty!"

"Yeah. I get that a lot. So I thought I may as well make money out of it."

"Well, I'm not surprised men like you. You're very pretty." She shrugs.

"I don't think so. It's just because I wear short skirts and I have big breasts. You must get lots of attention too."

"Not really. I don't wear short skirts."

"You don't need to, though. I bet you get chatted up all the time."

"No, I don't."

"I don't believe you", she giggles. I'm dying to ask her about the suicide attempt, but I don't want to upset her. But then again, she must have told dozens of people by now, so I bring it up as tactfully as I can. "My boyfriend dumped me. It was my fault really; I was a bitch to him. But I didn't mean to."

"Does he know you're here?"

"Yeah. If it was up to him I'd never leave this place."

"He must really hate you, to put you through this."

"He thinks the world is safer now I'm locked away."

"I think the world would be safer without most people in it. But I wouldn't count you in, you're a nice girl." I nearly faint as I finish my sentence. I just paid her two compliments in less than a minute! I'm so embarrassed,

I want to hide. I hate complimenting people. But she doesn't seem bothered, thankfully. She just smiles and looks away. What if I've embarrassed her as well, though? And what if she thinks I was coming on to her? Oh God. I have to find something to say to make up for it.

"Ah well, there are plenty of men around." I look around, pretending to check some of them out. "Anyone here you like?" She bites her lip.

"Can you keep a secret?"

"Sure."

"I'm kind of seeing Paul."

"Paul?"

"Yeah. We had sex yesterday."

"Sex? But ... Where?"

"Outside the Family Planning building, can you believe it?" No, I really can't. I thought I'd heard it all.

"But ... Didn't anyone see you?"

"No! Isn't that mad?"

"Yeah. That's ... unbelievable."

"It's kind of weird I suppose. It's quite ironic, doing it at the family planning! But we were really desperate. He'd been talking about it for days, so eventually, I gave in. You won't tell anyone, will you?"

"No, of course not. But ... Isn't he a bit old for you?"

"At least he's not fifty", she says looking at the bearded man. Then we both laugh.

"I suppose he's quite cute". It's a lie, but I felt obliged to say it.

"He is, isn't he?"

"Is it serious?"

"I don't know. Yesterday was the first time. But he's really nice."

"And he seems intelligent."

"He is. He always comes out with words and expressions I've never heard before. Like the other day, he said something like, "There's a circle inside each square.""

"What square?"

"I don't know."

"Huh. Maybe he makes things up to impress you."

"Maybe. And it works!"

"Well … that's good. As long as you're happy." I wish I meant it. But how can two people who have mental disabilities form a serious relationship together? He could be a complete psycho for all she knows. And so could she, actually.

"Is that your phone ringing?" She asks. I ended up charging my phone in the nurses' office, as Ali promised me he'd look after it. I hadn't noticed it was ringing. It's my mother. I cut her off. A second later she calls back, so I cut her off again.

"Have you got a stalker or something?"

"It's my mother."

"Oh. Does she know you're here?"

"No way. She'd think I'm trying to get people's attention or something."

"My father's like that. He's the one who brought me here."

"Really? What happened?"

"He found me unconscious, so he drove me to the hospital and asked them if they could keep me. I hate him. He blames me for him and my mum getting divorced."

"How can that be your fault?"

"I don't know. He's never liked me anyway."

"Same here. My parents have always preferred my sister."

"What's she like?"

"The opposite of me. Outgoing, beautiful, popular... She nearly died last week. She took some drugs and ended up in hospital."

"That's harsh. Is she OK?"

"I think so. But my mother blamed me for it. She said if I'd been around at her party she wouldn't have done it."

"That's bullshit. People do drugs because they want to. Even if she hadn't taken anything that night she would have some other time anyway. Don't beat yourself up about it. What was it she took?"

"Ecstasy I think."

"That's bad luck. Had she done it before?"

"I don't know. She tried to talk to me about it but I ignored her. I didn't realise she was planning to take drugs."

"What did she say?"

"She asked if I'd ever taken any. So I said no and changed the subject."

"Really? You've never taken drugs?"

"No, why? Have you?"

"Yeah, lots. Too many, actually. Until recently I couldn't watch TV because I was convinced it was talking to me."

"That's scary. Why do you take drugs? What's so great about them?" I'm intrigued.

"I don't know. You get high. You feel good. Everything is nice. You feel like the world is a great place and everyone loves you."

"See, I don't understand that. I'd rather hate and be hated genuinely than falsely loved because of some chemicals that will dissolve after a couple of hours."

"But those couple of hours are precious to me. When I'm on drugs, I'm happy. I forget how shit my life is. How much I hate myself. But my doctor told me if I didn't stop I could become like Lea."

"If you thought your TV was talking to you then yes, probably best to keep off them."

"I've been clean for weeks now. I'm going to try not to take anything when I come out."

"Good. You shouldn't. Even if it weren't for the voices, they damage your whole body", I say, probably sounding like an old textbook.

"I know. I used to have to take ice cold showers the day after pilling because my body was getting so hot. And one day I collapsed in the bath, I think I even convulsed. I had really weird nightmares about some monsters in a fairground; when I woke up it was like half an hour later, I was on the floor with slobber all over my mouth."

"And that didn't make you want to stop?"

"I tried to. But it's not that easy. Especially when most of your friends give you free pills all the time."

"Maybe you have the wrong friends. I wouldn't go near someone who tried to kill me."

"It's not like that. You can't understand if you've never been in that situation."

"My sister nearly died because someone gave her drugs. I don't think I'm being unreasonable."

"Yeah. I'm sorry. At least she's OK now, right? And hopefully she won't take anything ever again."

"I hope so." I feel like running to the loo and throw up. What if Jenny ends up like her? But there's no reason why she'd become anything that Sam is. My parents have given her everything. They couldn't show her more affection if they tried. I don't resent Sam … I feel rather sorry for her. I fear for her safety; I want her to be happy. I want to find her Dad and kill him. I want to find her ex boyfriend, and kill him too. And I want Paul to swear on his life that he'll look after her properly. I want to see Jenny and give her a hug. Tell her how much I'm sorry.

"Are you OK? I didn't mean to upset you or anything."

"No, don't worry. I'm fine. So … what are you going to do about Paul? Are you going to keep it a secret for long? Someone is bound to catch you if you keep shagging on the grounds, you know."

"Wouldn't that be bad? I wonder what they'd do. I bet we wouldn't be allowed out for weeks."

"Now that you mention it … How come I'm not allowed to go out?"

"Probably because you've just arrived. They have to know you before they can let you do things. I bet you're not even allowed to take any of the classes."

"What kind of classes?"

"Yoga, drama, stuff like that." That's so unfair. Not that I would take any classes but I'd like to be given the choice. I mean, what's there to do apart from sit on my arse all day watching TV, waiting for tea breaks and lunches and dinners? How am I supposed to get better with such a long amount of time on my hands to think about how crap everything is? It's a joke. What on earth are all the nurses for? All I've seen them do so far is give people pills, tell them off and sit in the lounge, supposedly writing on their pads but actually watching TV most of the time. I wonder what they write. I wonder what they get from someone staring at a big screen.

X: Flicks through channels = possible mania.

Y: Stares at screen silently = autism?

Z: Cries during Eastenders = depression.

"You've got a message." Sam says pointing at my phone again. "You really are in your own little world!"

"That's because I'm not used to it ringing."

"Really?" She giggles. "How do people get hold of you then?"

"They don't." It's from my mother.

"Hi, Melanie. Your sister is being discharged tomorrow. I was hoping you would come with us to pick her up. Can you let me know, your phone keeps cutting me off." I should be there. I should be picking her up myself. What am I going to tell my mother?

"Good news?"

"Not really. My sister's coming out of hospital tomorrow and I can't pick her up."

"Don't worry, you'll be out soon and you can see her then."

"Yeah but how am I supposed to justify the fact that I won't be there tomorrow?"

"I'm sure we can figure something out. I'll help you, I'm a good liar. Lea, are you OK?" Lea is sitting by herself, a couple of tables away from us. She's holding her head between her hands, crying and shaking. "Lea?"

"I'm OK." But she obviously isn't.

"What's wrong?" I ask. But she doesn't answer.

"She gets like that sometimes", Sam says matter of factly. A nurse is standing by the door. She looks at her briefly, then starts talking to Mourad.

"That is a lot of bread, dear. Make sure you eat it all, will you. Too much food gets wasted here."

"Is she taking the piss? She's more interested in bread waste than one of her patients being upset!" I cry.

"They don't give a shit." I get up and walk towards the nurse.

"Excuse me, I think Lea needs help."

"What's wrong with her?"

"I don't know! Surely that's for you to find out?"

"I don't think there's anything we can do. She does that sometimes."

"And you never do anything about it?"

"What can we do? She hears voices. I can't go inside her head and shut them up."

"So you're just going to stand here?"

"As I said, there's nothing we can do. Just go back to your table and ignore her." I don't need to; by the time I sit back down she's disappeared.

"Don't worry. She'll be OK", Sam says.

"But she must be so scared. All these noises in her head."

"I know. But there's not much we can do, apart from showing her that we care. And I'm sure she knows that."

"You're very mature for seventeen."

"I have to be. At seven I was already catching the bus on my own."

"Why?"

"Because my Mum didn't have time to drive me to school."

"But surely that's illegal?"

"I don't know. But we were in a small town and the drivers knew me, so it wasn't so bad", she says as though she was trying to defend her irresponsible mother. No wonder she ended up here so young; she didn't have a very good start in life, what with a mother who couldn't be bothered to take her to school and a father who blamed her for his divorce. I don't feel particularly loved but at least my parents didn't let me out on my own until I was twelve.

"I'm a Catholic, a Jew, a Muslim and a Pagan. I'm not gay, but if you are it doesn't matter", I hear behind me.

"This bloke is so annoying", Sam says. I turn around and see Jeff talking to the old knitting woman. "Is this like, his motto or something?"

"He's so freaky. I bet he's a rapist or something. I really want to see his notes."

"I'd love to see what the nurses write about me."

"You can. You just have to give them ten pounds." I laugh. "I'm not joking."

"What? You have to pay them to know what's wrong with you?"

"Yep."

"But ... that's ridiculous!"

"I know. But what's not ridiculous about this place? Apart from the food? Which, by the way, you should eat sometimes!"

"I do eat. I eat lots."

"Are you a vegetarian?"

"No, why?"

"I haven't seen you eat any meat."

"I don't eat it very often. It's too fattening." She shakes her head.

"You're so mad!"

"Well, yes ... I guess I am."

"Time to go upstairs!" The nurse shouts.

"Great. Four hours of TV until the next break."

"I can lend you a book or something if you like. My mum's picking me up soon; I'm spending the afternoon at home."

"Are you? How come?" I ask, feeling disappointed somehow. I enjoy her company.

"I'm allowed sometimes. My best mate's coming over, so we're going to get pissed!" I want to get pissed.

"I guess a book would be nice." She takes me to her room, where someone is asleep in the bed next to hers.

"That's all she ever does. She only gets up to eat and tap on the wall."

"Tap on the wall?"

"Yeah. It's quite funny. You'll probably see her do it soon. So, I've got these ... Or you can listen to some music if you want." She takes out a dozen CDs, all of them showing pictures of skulls, guns or long-haired men in tight clothes.

"I don't think I know any of these bands."

"It's heavy metal. What do you like?"

"Err... Aretha Franklin... Barry Manilow..."

"Oh my God. Are you eighty or something? I don't have any of those."

"Sam? Your mother's here. Is she still asleep?" The nurse from the canteen asks pointing at the tapping woman.

"Looks like it. I have to go, Mel. Take whatever you want." I look at the pile of books on her bed; I didn't think Shakespeare and Nietzsche went with Heavy Metal; but I guess I'm rather clueless when it comes to teenagers. For all I know my sister could be an ardent philosopher despite her tacky love for boy bands.

"Have I missed lunch?" Sam's roommate asks as she gets up.

"Yes, I'm afraid so."

"Did they come to get me?"

"I don't know, sorry. But if you tell them you were sleeping they'll probably give you something to eat".

She walks to the door and stops, standing right in front of it. Then she starts tapping. Left, right, left, and right again. She does it ten times, counting slowly and frowning, as though her movements required a high level of concentration. Then she goes away. I pick up the thinnest looking book and go to my room. I realise that I haven't rung my mother back, and think of a plan.

"What took you so long?", is the first thing she says when she picks up.

"Sorry, I was in a meeting. I didn't realise Jenny was coming out tomorrow. I'd love to pick her up but I'm in Bristol for a couple of days."

"Bristol? What are you doing in Bristol?"

"It's a work thing; I'm really sorry. But tell her I'll come to see her as soon as I'm back." But of course it's not good enough.

"Can't you tell them you have a family emergency?"

"No. If I had known about Jenny, I wouldn't have gone; but I was only told about this trip yesterday anyway. I can't leave now."

"So they only gave you a few hours notice?" She sounds suspicious.

"Yes. They're not very organised."

"I can see that. Well, if you can't, there's not much to do. I'll send Jenny your love, shall I?"

"Yes, please. And do tell her I will come over at the weekend." I hang up greatly relieved. I'm only hoping she's not going to ring the office to check up on me. I switch my phone off, deciding not to turn it back on until I come out.

"It's the end of the world. Soon. We're all going to die, you know", my second roommate shouts as she comes in. I briefly glance at her from the corner of my book and resume my reading. "Didn't you hear me?" she says, standing by my bed.

"Yes, I did."

"Don't you care?"

"Not really. I'm more interested in what happens to Macbeth right now."

"Why don't you care? Why aren't you scared? You're going to die too, you know! All of us!"

"And when's that going to happen then?"

"New Year's Eve. This year."

"Says who?"

"My mother. She sees things. She's always right."

"Really? And what room is she in?" But she doesn't get it. Although I was only half joking.

"I don't know! I can't see where she is, can I? I'm not a medium!" I sigh.

"Never mind."

"Why aren't you scared?" She repeats, looking horrified. "Are you a witch?"

"No, I'm not a witch. I'm just one of those people who either don't believe in the end of the world or aren't scared of it."

"Well, you'll be sorry. December the 31st. Don't say I didn't warn you."

"I won't." She goes out again, Mumbling to herself. I wonder where I'll be on New Year's Eve. I wonder if these people will still be here at Christmas. If their families will pick them up for the day or if they'll be stuck behind these walls. I hope Sam will go home. I wonder what Christmas would have been like if Jenny had died. An awful one, no doubt. Like most kids, it used to be my favourite time of the year; but after my sister was born I wasn't the centre of attention anymore - which at the time, funnily enough, I enjoyed - and I couldn't understand why a child before the age of at least three or four should get any presents, let alone a dozen, as they wouldn't know what they were anyway and would certainly not remember them later. But, no, Jenny had to get the best things, the shiniest and most expensive ones and I was left with whatever my parents could afford once they'd get all her stuff. Of course, now, it's irrelevant. But when I was growing up, for weeks before and after Christmas, I resented her. And later, I realised that really, it wasn't her fault, and the anger went towards my parents instead.

"Are you Linda?" the Turkish woman shouts as she comes in.

"No. I'm Melanie", I answer dryly. I hate being disturbed when I'm reading.

"Do you know who Linda is?"

"No."

"There's a phone call for her."

"I don't know who she is." She shrugs, sits on her bed and starts playing with her hair. "Weren't you looking for someone?"

"What?"

"You were just looking for Linda", I say trying to keep calm.

"Oh. I don't know who she is."

"You just said there was a phone call for her. Shouldn't you try to find her?"

"What?" If it was my book, and I knew for sure she wasn't a psychopath, I'd throw it at her.

"Never mind." But as well as playing with her hair, she starts singing in Turkish again. "Sorry, can you be a bit quieter? I'm trying to read." But she ignores me. Never mind if she's a psychopath, if I have to listen to her, I'll end up one as well. "Hey! Shut up, I'm trying to read!" She stops instantly, and gives me a horrified look.

"Rea, have you just picked up the phone and left it again? How many times have I asked you not to answer the phone when it rings? Who was it for?" someone asks, but I don't bother looking up to see who.

"L … L … Lin … da."

"Linda? There's no Linda here. You mean Lea?"

"Yes!"

"For fuck's sake, don't do that again!" the woman shouts as she storms out. I wonder how many fights they get here. There must be lots. Thinking of which, I never saw that drunken woman again. I hope they didn't kill her. Could they do that? I suppose they could easily pretend it was suicide. But I doubt anyone would buy it, since they won't even lend us a phone charger.

"Why are you here?" the Turkish woman asks. For crying out loud! I thought she'd got the message. Why is she trying to talk to me? I pretend I didn't hear, so she repeats herself.

"Because I'm mad. Can I read my book now?"

"I'm coming out soon. They're discharging me." She's having a laugh. Or maybe they've realised she was a hopeless case. But I fear for anyone coming across her.

108

How could they let someone like her out on the loose? She pees in her bed, for God's sake! I wonder how many of the mad people you see on the streets or on buses come from places like this one. And what makes the people working here think that they're fit enough to be left to live their lives without any supervision? Maybe they just give up on them after a while. I'd do anything for them to give up on me now; I feel like I haven't been out for weeks. It can't be healthy, you need natural air. It's so sunny out there. Sam can happily shag right outside the Family Planning building, but I can't take a walk in the park. I'm exasperated. It's hard to admit but I almost feel worse than I did before I came here. What keeps me from losing it completely is the realisation that 99% of the people here are probably worse off than I am. At least I'm not haunted by voices and I don't piss in my bed.

By the time dinner comes, Sam's still not back. I sit with Paul and he tells me about his plans to become a physics teacher, "to impress Sam". He seems to really care about her. It's quite sweet. Then I stick my clothes in the washing machine again and go watch TV in the smoking room, so that only a few people see me wear the stupid pink flowery pyjamas. I find myself waiting for Sam, but she doesn't come. A very short woman in her fifties, who seems more like an elf than a human, invites me to the party she's "throwing" at the weekend. "It's to celebrate the fact that I got my new glasses! We're all going to pretend we're children, it's going to be so much fun! I'm going to be a six year-old who doesn't want to wear her glasses!"

"I won't be there, I'm being discharged in a couple of days."

"Really? That's such a shame! There'll be food and drinks, obviously soft drinks, because we're all kiddies, aren't we! And music. Oh, and everyone has to have a nickname! I'll be Cupcakes! And you could be …"

"I'm quite happy with Melanie, thanks."

"Yeah, leave her alone, Chris. She's not interested", a young black woman intervenes. Chris shrugs and goes away. "Don't listen to her, she's off her head. I'm Melissa."

"Hi."

"You're Sam's friend?" Her friend? Is that what she says about me? That's nice.

"Y … Yes, that's right. Do you know her well?"

"Kind of. We've been here for nearly as long. I can't believe they're already discharging you. D'you know how lucky you are?"

"Yeah, I guess I am. Have you got long left?"

"I'm not sure. Three, four weeks maybe. I'm hoping less. This place is driving me crazy."

"I'm glad you said that, I thought it was just me!"

"People like us and Sam don't belong here. We should be in a different ward."

"Why are you here?"

"I went out with this guy for like, three years and he treated me like shit. Worse than a dog. He'd starve me, wouldn't let me leave the house if he didn't feel like it; he'd beat me up when I tried to stand up for myself."

"That's horrible. What made you stay with him for so long?"

"He kept telling me no one would want me because I wasn't worth anything. That he was the only one who would ever love me. And that if I left him he would find me and kill me."

"Jesus. That's frightening."

"So one day I went a bit mad and I got sent here. I'm glad to be honest, because I know he can't touch me here."

"What will happen when you leave though?"

"I don't know. He's been calling my mum and everything. He said if she didn't tell him where I was he'd kill her too. So the police got involved and now he's not allowed anywhere near us. But I don't know how long that's going to keep him away for."

"But you don't want to go back to him, do you?"

"No way. I should have left ages ago. But I was too scared."

"That's understandable."

"They said when I come out they're going to help me find my own place and look for work. I can't wait."

"Really? They can do that?"

"Yeah. That's about the only thing this place is good for."

"So what's up with that Chris woman?"

"God knows. She's always on about being children and fairy tales and all that crap. And she thinks a couple of bags of crisps and some Diet Coke make a party. She's in her own little world. What are you planning to do when you come out?"

"Have a bath ... change clothes ... go to work, if I haven't been sacked."

"Why would you get sacked?"

"Cause I'm crap at it. And I told them I'd twisted my ankle, but they'll probably notice I'm fine. Well, physically fine at least."

"So you haven't told them you were here?"

"No way!"

"Why?"

"Why? Because ... it's embarrassing."

"You shouldn't think like that. Being depressed is really common, you know."

"It's not only that. I'm not sure how what they'd make of the suicide attempt. They might think I could do it again, they might think I'm unstable."

"Well ... Yes. To be honest, you probably are. But they can't get rid of you for that. What have you got to lose anyway? If you think they'll sack you because you lied, you may as well tell them the truth."

"I guess." She's probably right, but how could I tell them? Maybe they wouldn't be too surprised, they've probably always thought I was mad. I wonder what counselling would be like. Naomi would be pleased if she knew. "I told you so!" she'd probably say with a big smile on her face. But there's no way I'm going. The thought of someone getting paid to listen to my problems, to hear how shit my life is and how bad I feel makes me cringe. I'd rather keep it all in, thank you very much. How do these people live with themselves? You open your heart, probably have a few sobs here and there, tell them things you've told no one before, and when time is up you're asked to leave the rest to the next session and pay them! And what are you supposed to do until the next session? The counsellor moves on to their next patient, and when their shift is over, they put it all behind them, have their nice little family life, whilst the patient is left to feel alone and miserable for a week.

"You look very thoughtful."

"I'm just wondering what good counselling can really do. It doesn't appeal to me at all."

"Are you going to be referred somewhere?"

"The doctor said so. But I don't think it's for me. For one thing, I can't afford it."

"I doubt they'd make you pay. They'd probably refer you somewhere on the NHS."

"Really? You don't always have to pay?"

"No, not on the NHS. Didn't you know?"

"No. I'd never thought about it." Free therapy. That's good. Well, for people who need it, of course? That doesn't mean I do.

I go to bed early, hoping I'll fall asleep quickly but I lay awake for hours, not just because of the snores of the Turkish bitch, but also because my mind won't shut up; work, Jenny, my parents, even Naomi and Simon. I suppose the good thing about being here, apart from not spending any money, is that I don't have to see any of them. Although it would be nice to have some form of normal company right now.

****

The next couple of days are the longest I've ever had to live. All I can think of is going out and drinking. I feel numb, alienated and more stressed than ever. The night before my discharge, I don't sleep; thankfully Sam is an insomniac too, and as she got back from her mum's late and drunk, she's not allowed to go out for a week, so I sit on her bed and we talk for hours; I never thought I'd say that of a teenager, but I think I really like her. She says she'll miss me, and even suggests that we keep in touch! When morning comes, I'm told I'll have to wait until after lunch; so, with a knot in my stomach, I wait. In my head, I make a list of all the things I'm going to do: bath, wash my hair, change clothes, go online, possibly throw up (I think I've put on half a stone since I've been here. How is that possible?), rent films, call Jenny, maybe even Naomi … although I haven't made up my mind yet. When time finally comes, I hug Sam, Lea and Melissa and follow the nurse along the corridors. I take a last look around me; the yellow walls, the muddy lino floors, the cramped rooms.

"There you are." I stare at the door with great apprehension. I haven't gone through it for five days. I've been looking forward to this moment since the minute I got here, but now that the time has come, I'm scared. As though I belonged here more than out there. "Have you changed you mind, dear? Go on, off you go!" So I do. I walk down the stairs, through more corridors, open another door and I'm out. I walk past half a dozen different wards, The Willows, The Chestnuts, Halliwick, until I finally find the path that takes me back into the "real" world. It's so hot, so sunny, so … alive! There are so many places I want to go to, so many things I want to do, I don't know where to start. I go home to take a bath and then I lie down in front of the TV. From time to time,

I find myself expecting a nurse to come in and announce the tea break! I make some dinner, then turn my PC on and to my astonishment, I find an email from Simon.

"Hi, Melanie. I just wanted to apologise for last Saturday. I know I came across as an arsehole, but I guess that's because I was trying to impress you. I realise now I didn't go the right way about it. Can you forgive me? Maybe we could meet up again before I leave. I hope you can find it in your heart to give me a second chance."

I read these lines about ten times. Why would he want to see me again? He must be bored. If he really cared he would have phoned me. I just want to forget I ever met him. I don't want to have to think about that day. Does he realise I nearly died because of him? Even if I wanted to see him, which I don't, it'd be too late, because he's leaving in a couple of days. But I don't want to ignore him, I want him to fully understand how much I resent him.

"Simon,

You're a fucking wanker and I hate you!"

That probably sounds too childish.

"Simon,

Do you realise I tried to kill myself because of you?"

I don't think he needs to know that. It'd only boost his ego.

Simon,

I'm glad that you realised things didn't go well. I was very disappointed; but maybe it's my own fault for expecting too much of someone I had never met before. I've had a lot of time to think since that day, and in a way, I'm grateful it happened, because it made me understand a few things. I don't think we should meet again. What would be the point? You live on the other side of the world. I'm not sure we should talk online either; I wouldn't know if I were talking to the real you or a product of your wide imagination. Good luck with everything.

****

Phil is cross. He's very cross. "This is a very unprofessional behaviour, Melanie. Did you think we wouldn't notice? So go on, tell me. What have you really been doing for the past five days?"

"I … I was in a mental hospital."

"A mental hospital?" He grins. "What on earth were you doing in a mental hospital?"

"I was ill. I became depressed. I … I tried to kill myself. So I had to stay in a mental hospital. They wouldn't let me go." He stares at me with his little eyes, still grinning.

"Well, I can't say I'm surprised! I knew there was something wrong with you."

"I … I feel better now. If it had been up to me, I wouldn't have spent a single night there."

"And if it had been up to me, they would have kept you."

"What … What do you mean?"

"I'm sorry Mel, but we can't have you here. I don't understand why they let you out, really. But anyway, as I said, I don't think you're fit enough to work with us."

"But ... I'm fine, really, I am!"

"I knew making you supervisor was a mistake. If we kept you, what kind of image would we be projecting of ourselves? We can't have loonies here! Go now. And please, don't talk or approach anyone on your way out."

OK, this would be the worse case scenario. But it could happen. I won't know until I tell him the truth. Maybe I should just not say anything and wait to see if he mentions the doctor's certificate. Yes, I'll do that.

"Melanie! Back with us at last. How are you?"

"Hi Phil. I feel better, thanks. Where do you want me?" I try to sound as calm as I can.

"Can you just pop into my office for a sec? I'll give you an update on what's been happening."

"Sure."

"Sit down. Right ..." He plays with his fingers silently, raising his eyebrows from time to time. "Before we start, there's something I've been quite concerned about. You see, a few days ago I got a phone call from your mother. She was under the impression we'd sent you to Bristol. I don't know where she got that from. She didn't seem to be aware that you'd hurt your ankle." I knew it. Why did she have to call them? She was checking on me. She's such a cow. I hate her! "Why would she think you were in Bristol? We don't even have an office there!" Melissa's right. If I'm going to lose my job I might as well be honest.

"Because I told her."

"But ... Why would you do such a thing?"

"Because ... Because I didn't really twist my ankle."

"I don't understand." I can feel my eyes getting heavy and wet. "You lied?"

"Yes. I did."

"But why? If you wanted to take some time off, you should have just asked!"

"It wasn't like that. Something ... Something happened. Something I couldn't help."

"You're going to have to explain yourself more clearly." He says in a drier voice.

"I ... I wasn't feeling very well. So I ... I tried to ... commit suicide. But someone found me and I was sent to a mental hospital. I wasn't allowed to leave until yesterday. I'm really sorry." I can't contain the tears any longer. I cry like I haven't cried for a very long time. I'm embarrassed, ashamed to admit to such a weakness. I daren't looking at him, but I can sense the horror in his eyes.

"My God. I had no idea. I'm sorry to hear that, Melanie. Awfully sorry."

"And I'm sorry for wasting your time. I may as well go now."

"What do you mean, go?"

"You going to sack me, aren't you?"

"Of course not! Why would I do such a thing?"

"Because ... Because I lied and I'm dreadful at this job anyway!"

"Why on earth would you think that? As I said to you before, you're one of our best employees! And there is no way I would sack you for what happened last week. I just feel really bad for not noticing that you were feeling this way." He hands me a tissue. I still can't look at him. "I don't know what to say … If you're not ready to come back, why don't you take some time off? Go on holiday somewhere. It might do you some good."

"No, I can't. But you don't have to keep me. I would understand if you didn't."

"Please, don't think that. You will always be welcome here. Let me think… Maybe you could take it easy today, and come back tomorrow morning. It's very quiet anyway so there wouldn't be much for you to do right now."

"I … I guess so."

"Good. Now, you take care of yourself and I'll see you in the morning. And if you ever need to talk, whatever it is, you know where I am. Don't be embarrassed about anything. Alright?"

"Yes. Thank you." I want to jump out of my chair and hug him. Did he really mean that? I think so. Maybe I was wrong about him. He's given me a day off! I could do with it, to be honest. I need time to recover from everything, including this. I'm so glad I haven't lost my job. I don't know what I would have done if I had. So, what now? Maybe I could do some shopping; I haven't bought myself anything for ages. I could get some new software for my PC or some videos. I wish I could have a pet. But even if the landlord let me, it couldn't be a dog or a cat because my flat is too small. A rabbit would chew all my cables and I'd probably lose anything smaller. I bet I could easily vacuum it up. As a child the only animal I was ever allowed was a goldfish; my mother used to say I'd kill anything bigger. But fish are so boring; you can't do anything with them. As an alternative, I go to my regular PC store and buy Petz II, as it's on sale for only £2.99. I pick a gorgeous virtual ginger kitten and spend most of the afternoon playing with it. I wish Nam could see it … She loves cats. I wonder how she is. Maybe I should call her. What's the worst that can happen? She'd tell me to get lost and put the phone down on me. Maybe it'd be easier if I spoke to her face to face. At least then she'd have to hear me out. I can't go to her flat though, what if her boyfriend's there? It'd be so embarrassing. I need to see her alone. I could go to her uni … I'm sure she said she was taking some other weird summer class.

I wait by the gate, whilst hundreds of students walk in an out, and I wonder if I'll manage to spot her and if I'll have to wait hours before she comes out. Thankfully, after only 20 minutes she appears … and she doesn't seem too pleased to see me.

"What are you doing here?"

"I wanted to see you."

"Why?" I can't tell if she's annoyed or worried about what I might say or do.

"I needed to talk to you. Can we go somewhere?"

"I'm really busy. I've got an essay to write for tomorrow." She's lying. Knowing her, she would have finished it at least a week ago.

"Please. Just five minutes." She hesitates.

"Fine. Five minutes."

We sit in the nearest café; it hasn't been long since last time I saw her, but she looks a completely different person. Her hair is no longer dry and fizzy, but straight and silky; she's wearing eye shadow and her clothes are much tighter than they used to be. I wonder if George is behind all this.

"So, what have you got to say?"

"I'm sorry." She rolls her eyes and sighs. "I mean it. You were right … I was selfish. I've been thinking lots." She stays silent for a while, playing with her cup.

"I've been thinking too. Thing is, I don't see the point in being friends with you, Melanie. I mean, let's face it. The only thing we had in common was the fact that we didn't have anyone else. But what happened last time I saw you made me realise that I shouldn't rely on just one person and certainly not taking everything they say as the gospel. So I've made new friends. I didn't think it would be easy, but you know what? All you have to do is be nice to people. And I am a nice person. I've always been! But somehow you'd managed to convince me it wasn't worth it, that the whole world was crap and that I'd always be as sad as you. But I'm not like you! I never was! Haven't you got anything to say? No, that's right, you never face up to anything. The only reason you're here is that you didn't have anyone else to moan to!" I know she's right. Of course she is. That's why I don't argue. I finish my coffee, say goodbye and go back home. I feel sad, and hurt… we were friends for a long time. I really wanted to tell her about the hospital, but I just couldn't bring myself to it. I knew this would happen, sooner or later. Best to end it this way than to keep on having stupid arguments like the one we had last time, I suppose. I know I did the right thing by trying to patch things up, though. If I hadn't done it I would have regretted it later. I've wasted so much time being miserable and hating everyone; maybe I've missed out on a lot of good things, and good people. But it's so much easier to see the worst in someone. Well, I'm going to put it all behind me now. I can make friends, like everyone else. I did at the hospital and I can do it again. It's not my fault I haven't met the right people yet! I used to be nice; I wasn't born unfriendly and miserable. Until I met Naomi, I was always people's "second best friend"; like a replacement for when the actual best friend wasn't around. And if I were ever close enough to someone to feel that I might actually like them and that they might like me, they'd change school or move abroad. So of course when I started hanging out with Naomi, I couldn't believe my luck. Now, I feel vacant. I have a sudden urge to eat. Bread, yoghurt, cheese, chocolate, pizza, I need them all. But there's nothing in my fridge: just milk, vegetables and orange juice. Why haven't I got any food!

NHS

PSYCHOLOGICAL THERAPIES SERVICE

Halliwick Psychotherapy Department

St Mary's Hospital

St Mary's Road

London N14 8TH

Tel: 020 8534 7107

October 1st, 2002

Dear Ms Stevenson,

Mr Schoenberg, Psychiatrist at the North Middlesex Hospital, has asked me to offer you an appointment for assessment for psychological therapy. Could you please come and see me in the Psychotherapy Department at St Mary's Hospital, on Friday, October 12th?

I would be grateful if you could confirm with my secretary on the above number that this time is convenient for you. Please note that if we do not hear from you by Monday, October 8th, we will assume that you do not wish to take up the appointment.

With thanks for you co-operation.

Yours sincerely,

Chrissie Da Costa

So soon? I was hoping they'd forget about me. And I was never told I'd have to go back to that hospital! I don't know if I should. I don't see the point. It'd be a total waste of time. And it would be so strange to be back there. It's free, apparently, but still. I don't think so. But I'm not working that day. Oh well, maybe, if I haven't got anything else planned. They can't expect me to move my life around for them, can they? I wonder what we'd talk about; what they'd offer me. I suppose there's no harm in going. Especially if it is free, like Melissa said. But I won't tell anyone. It's bad enough that Phil knows. I hope he won't use it as an excuse to patronise me. I lie on my bed and stare at the wall for a while. Things are changing. I don't like change.

****

"Ms Stevenson? Come through." I follow Chrissie along the corridors, into a small office. She waits until I sit down and look as though I'm ready to listen before she starts to speak.

"My name is Chrissie, and I'm a senior psychological nurse here, at St Mary's." She's short, chubby, with huge curls and freckles all over her face. She can't be older than twelve. "As you probably know, you have been referred here by doctor Brown, whom you met in the Lordship ward. Did he tell you much about us?" I shrug.

"No. Just that he'd pass me on to some counsellor."

"Can you tell me about the reasons you were taken to North Middlesex and here at St Mary's?"

"I would have thought they'd have told you themselves."

"But I would like to hear it from you." I sum it up as briefly as I can. I don't want to have to think about it again. "And why did you have those suicidal thoughts?" I shrug again.

"I don't know. I felt sad."

"Had something happened to make you feel that way?" I take a deep breath. I don't want to answer. I knew I would have to talk about this and I didn't want to. She doesn't say a word, so we both sit in silence. She's looking at me, and it makes me feel even more tense. After what feels like hours, she finally speaks.

"You don't have to answer at this stage if you don't want to." At this stage? What does that mean? That later they'll force the answers out of me? I can't be bothered to argue now.

"OK."

"How do you feel about counselling?"

"I don't know."

"Do you personally feel that you need counselling?"

"Maybe. I guess."

"What makes you think that you might need it?" I giggle, without really intending to.

"Because I was told so."

"By whom?"

"Friends. People at the hospital."

"And what do you think?"

"Like I said. Maybe." She hasn't stopped staring at me.

"What do you think a place like this can offer you?"

"I'm not with you."

"What do you expect from a therapy programme?" I laugh again.

"I don't know really. That you fix me?"

"What do you think needs fixing in you?" All these questions! It's too much effort. I can't bear to think about all this.

"I thought it was your job to tell me?"

"Not exactly. My job is to help you get better, but you have to want to be helped first. Do you?"

"Yes." Of course I do, I want to say. Why the hell would I be here otherwise? I hate her already.

"OK. Then I'll tell you about what we can offer you here. We currently have a programme called Intensive Outpatient Psychotherapy. It consists of two therapy sessions a week, one is a fifty minute individual session with a therapist, the other is an hour and a half group session. There will be five of you and I will be mediating it."

"By group session, do you mean that I'd have to sit with a bunch of people and hear them talk about how crazy they are?"

"You will be interacting with each other. You can talk about anything you like and comment on what the others say." I giggle in shock.

"And what would be the point of that?"

"You get to meet people who may share the same problems as you; it helps not feeling alone, knowing that others are going through what you are."

"Sorry, but I find it hard enough talking to you. I really don't see myself telling a group of strangers my life story."

"You won't have to discuss anything you don't want to. It's always difficult in the first sessions, but gradually people start to open up."

"I don't need opening up, I just want someone to tell me what's wrong with me and fix it!"

"These things take time and a lot of effort. It's not like fixing a car. It's an eighteen month programme, and ..."

"Eighteen months?"

"Yes. Do you think it's too much?"

"Of course I do! That's a year and a half of my life wasted!" She doesn't react; she still has the same vacant expression on her face.

"So you consider therapy as a waste of time?"

"I don't know yet. But eighteen months is a really long time."

"As I said, these things take time. Maybe you could give it a thought and come back to me with your decision?"

"And what if I don't want this?"

"Then we would have to refer you somewhere else. But the waiting lists can be very long and here you would be able to start straight away. This programme has proven to be very effective.

We leave it at that. Group therapy? What a joke. I want to laugh, but somehow I can't help my eyes watering. I have to share an hour and a half of my life every week with some strangers who are probably going to hate me straight away and make me feel worse about myself! And what for? How will I know that I'm not wasting my time? Even if I wanted to go, Phil would probably not allow me to take all this time off. Why did I open my mouth? All I had to do was say I was fine and she would have left me alone. I need to relax. I buy a couple of bottles, light some candles and turn my computer on, when someone knocks on the door. Who on earth could it be? I don't want to answer. But then last time I ignored it someone ended up at the morgue.

"Hello? Is anybody home?" I hear a woman say behind the door. I sigh and get up to open it and I'm faced with a skinny, bleached young boy. He's wearing a tight white t-shirt and an even tighter pair of jeans. "Hi there! I'm James, your new neighbour!" He presents me with his hand, so I shake it. It feels soft and silky. A typical gay man.

"I'm ... Melanie."

"Hello, Melanie! I've just moved upstairs and I thought I should introduce myself to everyone here!"

"You live at number 5?"

"That's right!" I thought it might take months for that flat to be rented again, given what happened in it. I wonder if there's still blood on the carpet. "I heard someone got killed up there!"

"Yes."

"Did you know them?"

"Not really."

"It's tragic, isn't it?" He says tapping his fingers against his cheek.

"Yes. It is."

"Apparently the landlord had to slash the rent because of all the bad publicity!"

"Well that's good for you then."

"You bet!" I really want to get rid of him, but I'm also dying to know what it's like upstairs now.

"Was there any blood or broken things in there?"

"No, it was all pristine! Bit of a shame in a way, it would have been quite interesting to see it the way it was. People turn green when I tell them I live on a crime scene! They say I'm mad, I suppose I must be!" By his looks and loudness I bet he's the kind of person who plays hideous pop music at three in the morning and brings back a different bloke every night. That's all I need right now. I don't have anything against gays, but they always seem so cheerful and hyper. It's exasperating. "So, where are the good bars around here? I'm new to the area."

"Oh, I don't know. I don't go out much."

"Really? Well in that case, we'll investigate together!"

"Y … Yeah. Sure." Over my bloody dead body.

"Fantastic!" He cries, clapping his hands. Does he think I'm going to be his best friend or something? "I'd better go to work, but I'll see you very soon!"

"Yeah. Nice meeting you." I close the door as he leaves. I surprise myself for not telling him to get lost straight away; my people skills are obviously improving.

NHS

PSYCHOLOGICAL THERAPIES SERVICE

Halliwick Psychotherapy Department

St Mary's Hospital

St Mary's Road

London N15 3TH

Tel: 020 8534 7101

14th October 2002

Dear Ms Stevenson,

Further to our meeting on 12th October, I have pleasure in confirming your admission into our Outpatient intensive Therapy programme. The hours will be every Tuesday from 13:00 until 14:30 for Group Therapy, and 10:00 until 10:50 every Thursday for Individual Sessions, which will be with Mr John Bergman. Your programme will start on Tuesday, 23rd October. If you cannot keep this appointment, please telephone the receptionist on the number indicated.

Yours sincerely,

Chrissie Da Costa

I'm nervous. I shouldn't be, it's only my sister, for Christ's sake. But that's the problem. What if she doesn't want to see me? What if my mother has managed to convince her that it was my fault? I'd never get over it. Yes, we have as much in common as a fish and a bicycle, but she's my flesh and blood. If she had died, part of me would have gone with her. I'm welcomed with a cold and blunt "Hello" from my mother. She seems surprised to see me, as though she'd been hoping that I'd changed my mind and not turned up. We managed not to mention the work incident when we were on the phone, but I fear she might bring it up any moment now, so I go straight to the point.

"Is she in her room?"

"Yes. She's been waiting for you for hours."

"But I'm ten minutes early?" She takes a few seconds to think of what to reply.

"Yes, well, she thought you might not come after all." I walk up the stairs quickly, to spare myself as much hassle as I possibly can. I knock on her door, holding my breath.

"Yeah?"

"It's me, Melanie." The door opens quickly; it's as though she'd been posted behind it.

"Melanie! Hi!" She greets me with a smile and a hug. I hug her back and we stand in each other's arms for a few seconds. Then she closes her door and we sit on her bed.

"So ... How are you?" As I say it, I giggle nervously, and so does she.

"I'm OK. I am, really. It was weird at first, mainly when I woke up in the hospital. I thought I was dreaming, or having a nightmare, rather. Especially because the first thing I saw was Mum's face!" I laugh, but at the same time my eyes water.

"She was really worried. So was dad. And so was I."

"I'm really sorry. I didn't mean to scare you. Sarah told me it was safe."

"Did Sarah give you the drugs?"

"Yeah. But she does it every weekend and nothing's ever happened to her."

"How many times have you done this?"

"That was the first time."

"But why did you do it?"

"I … I wanted to feel nice. Feel different. Sarah told me drugs made her happy."

"But … Aren't you happy?"

"Not really."

"But you're young and beautiful, you have all those friends and mum and dad love you … You have every reason to be happy."

"It's not that easy though, is it? Sometimes I feel like I don't fit in with anyone. And mum … Ever since you left, she's been unbearable."

"What do you mean?"

"She blames herself for you leaving; she knows she didn't give you enough attention. So she's constantly on my case, because she's scared I'm going to take off too. And I hate her for letting you go."

"Really?"

"I hated you at first. I felt like you'd abandoned me. But then I realised it wasn't my fault. Or at least I hoped it wasn't."

"Oh darling, of course not. I left because … I needed my space. My freedom."

"That's why I admire you. You've always been so independent."

"You admire me?"

"Yeah. I always have. I've always wanted to be like you." I never thought I'd hear her say that.

"But … why? What's so special about me?"

"You're … you!"

"Exactly. How could you want to be like that?" I'm shaking. I don't want her to turn into me. I want her to be nice. Happy. Not a bloody mental freak.

"Jenny, there's something I have to tell you." She looks at me attentively, which makes me feel self-conscious.

"You look so serious!" She says half laughing. Just as I open my mouth again, her phone suddenly rings.

"Sorry. Just a sec. Hello? Hiya. No I can't, my sister's here. Yeah, bye. What were you saying?"

"Nothing really. You know, you can stay at my place some time, if you still want to come to London."

"Do you mean it? Oh, thank you Mel, thank you so much! I'd love to. When can I come?"

"Whenever you want. Obviously not on a school day."

"Of course not! Let's think … I've got a friend's birthday party on next Saturday and the week after I'm going to Spain for ten days …"

"Spain? What are you doing in Spain?"

"It's a school thing. I study it, remember? We're going there to practise the language I suppose. So maybe after that?"

"Sure. Just remind me nearer the time. By the way, you're not planning to take anything at that party, are you?"

"No. I'm not planning on taking anything ever again."

"Good. Now … Do you fancy a trip to the shopping centre?"

"Are you serious? Of course!"

We go into every shop; she looks at everything; but this time, I make the effort of not arguing. I actually enjoy myself. I buy her a top, then we sit in a cafe and I listen to her talking about school and a guy she likes. She asks for my advice, which I struggle to give her, but in the end she seems satisfied. I go home with the feeling that I've finally bonded with my sister.

Chapter 5

I shouldn't have come. Why am I here? I could still go. I could get up and tell the receptionist I've forgotten to do something. Or I could just not say anything; it doesn't matter to her whether I'm here or not.

"Melanie? Would you like to come through?" Shit. Too late. Chrissie takes me into a larger room than last time, where four people are sat in a circle. I have to walk past all of them to find an empty chair, next to a girl dressed all in black, in the same style as Sam. She's wearing a hooded top that says "Protected by witchcraft". I wonder if she'd try to cast a spell on me if I pissed her off.

"So, this is Melanie. Maybe you should all introduce yourselves to her." Chrissie says; she looks at the girl next to me, as if to say, "You can start."

"I'm Rachel. Am I supposed to say anything else?"

"You can say whatever you want", Chrissie replies.

"I'm Rachel", she repeats.

"Hi", I answer.

"I'm Renee", says the girl next to her. She's wearing office type clothes; a plain cream top and Next-like black trousers. If I saw her in the streets, I'd never think she was mad.

"I'm Adam."

"And I'm Caroline." Caroline is obviously at least twenty years older than the rest of them. The bloke is tall, and looks like a muscled version of Ewan McGregor in Train Spotting.

"Maybe someone could summarise what we have been discussing these past few weeks", Chrissie says after an awkward silence. They all look at each other and seem unsure or maybe scared of what to say. Rachel is the first to speak.

"Self harm. Depression. Suicide. Men. Women. Love. Hate." As she goes on into a catalogue of words, the others start to giggle. I think she's taking the piss.

"We talk pretty much about everything", Renee adds in as Rachel stops to catch her breath.

"How was your weekend, Caroline?" Rachel says, not aware, or probably ignoring the fact that Renee hadn't finished. "Did you see your sister?"

"Yes I did, thank you for asking. It was quite stressful. She criticised me a lot, for a change."

"What about?"

"The usual. I drink too much. I've put on weight again. I'm too negative."

"Did you tell her that it upsets you when she says these things?"

"She knows it. I think she enjoys nagging me."

"That's horrible, isn't it? Families are always a nightmare." Rachel concludes on their dialogue. I get the feeling she's the dominant one. Probably an attention seeker. And I can tell she's going to annoy me a lot.

"Have you got any brothers and sisters, Melanie?"

"I have a younger sister."

"Do you get on with her?"

"Yeah. We're fine."

"You're lucky. I don't get on with mine either" Rachel says, shrugging.

"I wouldn't say I'm lucky. We've had our ups and downs."

"I don't think any of us are lucky. That's why we're here, isn't it?" They go on talking about their parents and siblings and I spend more time looking at the clock above Chrissie's head than listening and taking part in their dull reflection on whether you have to love your family just because they share your blood. Adam is the only one who has said less than me.

"We do have to finish now", Chrissie breaks off at 4:30pm sharp. She gets up and leaves first, and I follow straight after.

When I get back to my flat, I find a note from James under the door.

"Hey Mel! Fancy a drink tonight? Gimme a call!"

I can't believe I've only met this guy once and he's already giving me his phone number. I could be a psycho stalker for all he knows! I suppose if I wanted to stick to my resolutions, I should call him and go out. But I don't know if I could spend an evening with him without getting homicidal thoughts into my head. I could make up a polite excuse; but then, if I'm going to try and make friends I have to start somewhere. I dial his number slowly, hoping that he won't pick up. Thankfully, it's switched off, so I leave a quick message on his voicemail (part of me was tempted to give him a fake number but I decided against it). He calls me back soon after ... and before I know it, we're having cocktails in the nearest Whetherspoon's.

"Don't you love these pubs? A bit dull music wise obviously, since, hello! there isn't any, but it's the cheapest place to get pissed! Maybe once we're a bit tipsy we can move onto somewhere livelier?"

"I can't get drunk I'm afraid, I have to work tomorrow", I say, aware that I probably sound very boring.

"So have I darling! Don't you worry about a thing, you're safe with me!" He seems so excited and cheerful, it's kind of cute somehow. "So, what do you do, honey?" He asks before taking a sip of his Sex on the Beach.

"I work for a Market Research company. I'm a supervisor."

"So you boss people around and tell them off? Sounds fun!"

"It's not particularly fun; it's quite stressful, actually."

"Oh, why?"

"Because the people I supervise aren't always cooperative."

"Just tell them you'll sack them or give them a good spanking! You're the boss, Goddamit!" I giggle.

"What about you?"

"I work for Virgin."

"Really? That's … exciting."

"Yeah, it's great. Putting CDs on shelves requires a really high level of intelligence!"

"Is that all you do?"

"Nah, of course not. Sometimes I get to handle DVDs as well!" He says laughing.

"That's cool; I mean, it can be interesting, you get to know about all the latest releases and stuff …"

"No, it's boring as fuck! But I get a 20% discount!"

"Well, it's worth it then, isn't it?"

"Yeah, kind of. But that's not my life ambition of course, how sad would that be! It's just to pay the rent, until my career takes off."

"And what career would that be? This is delicious by the way", I say as I realise I've nearly emptied my glass already.

"I know, I love Sex on the Beach! Especially with a gorgeous tanned go-go boy! Well, my career ..." He puts his drink on the table, raises his hands up in the air and starts to sing "I will survive", in a high pitched voice that even Michael Jackson couldn't manage.

"Oh my God. You're amazing."

"Thank you, babes."

"Have you ever performed with an audience?"

"I do cabarets in gay bars; I dress up and all. But that's about it."

"That's a start, isn't it?"

"Yeah ... I'm thinking of applying for Pop Idol."

"You know, that's a really good idea."

"I don't think they're big on poofters though."

"They wouldn't reject you because of that! That's not allowed, is it? I mean, look at Will Young."

"I know, but he only came out after he'd won; most people who watched that show were spotty teenage girls and frustrated housewives ... they want to see people they can fantasise about."

"I watched it and I'm neither of those, I don't think. Although I have to say my aim is usually to laugh at the poor sods Simon Cowell takes the piss out of."

"And hopefully I wouldn't fall into that category or I'd have to kill myself. So maybe I should stick to cabaret for now. Another drink?"

"I'll get them!" Surprisingly, I'm enjoying this. It's a feeling I haven't had in a long time. I think I actually like James. We have a couple more cocktails, then move to a different bar. By the fifth drink, I'm rather drunk, and we start talking about men.

"I like mine beefy", he says and I can't help giggling again. I imagined him more with someone like Julian Clary. "The Grant Mitchell type, if you see what I mean."

"Is that the bald guy from Eastenders who shagged his wife's mother? I don't watch it but I remember reading about it in the papers."

"Yep, that's the guy."

"I don't understand soaps. Why do newspapers treat them like they're real life stories? I mean, do people not realise that they're just about as real as Milly Vanilly?"

"I guess the English are a bunch of sad low-lifers!"

"You're not wrong there. I wouldn't say I fancy Grant, though."

"So who's your dream guy then?"

"Err … I don't know really. Ewan McGregor maybe?"

"Yeah. Not bad. If you like ginger that is!" Strangely, as I said that, it wasn't actually him I pictured, but that Adam guy from the group. He was kind of cute.

"My God, I must be really drunk, I forgot about Kevin Spacey!"

"What about him?"

"He's … was … my dream guy!"

"You must be joking! Really? But he's like, fifty, isn't he?"

"I know! But I love him. Loved him … until today maybe? Oh, I don't know, I'm confused! You've got me too drunk!"

"Honey, you can't be drunk on five cocktails!" He makes big gestures with his hands and nearly hits a couple of people walking past. "Actually, I think I'm a bit pissed too!"

The rest of the evening is all mixed into a big blur. I don't remember leaving the bar, nor getting home. I know I hugged James goodnight and we said we should do it again soon, but that's as far as my memory goes. Surprisingly, I don't wake up with a hangover; I just worry that I might have said or done something embarrassing, like mentioning the therapy, or the mental hospital. But hopefully if I did, he was too drunk himself to remember now. Or maybe he wasn't drunk at all … maybe he was on fruit juice all night and pretended to be drunk, so he could get me to talk! But what for? Maybe he robbed me! Maybe I've given him my bank details or something! I mean, how will I know until I find that my account has been emptied? I check my wallet and thankfully all my cards are there; but I phone the bank and change my security codes, just in case.

The next day, I meet my therapist; my first impression of him is a better one than of Chrissie, but I still have my reservations. As I thought and feared, he asks me why I think I'm in therapy, what I want out of it and whether I mind him being a man, which until now I hadn't even thought of. So I say "no", because I don't want to offend him and also because I don't dislike men any more than women; at least men don't make me feel inferior … just vulnerable. The fifty minutes go quicker than I had expected; I actually find myself frustrated at the fact that I don't have time to say all I wanted to say. Funnily, he concludes the session with the same line as Chrissie, "We do have to finish now". It makes me wonder if they've been instructed to do that. In a way, I was hoping Phil wouldn't let me have the time off, because it would have given me an excuse not to go. "You have been given the chance to do something about your issues; you should take it", is what he'd said. But after two more weeks of therapy, I struggle to see the point of it; Rachel always seems to be the centre of attention in the group, interrupting everyone and monopolizing the discussions; and my sessions with John are too short to get anything out of them. After the end of the fourth group session, I'm ready to give up; but as I walk out of the room, I feel a tap on my shoulder. As I turn around, Renee says in a whisper, "Do you fancy coming for a drink with us?" I'm so surprised that it takes me a few seconds to form an answer.

"Err … Sure." I don't know why I said that; my mouth worked quicker than my brain. Why on earth would I want to go drinking with them?

"We usually go to a pub after the group. But we didn't want to ask you just when you started, we didn't know how you'd react, you see. We're not supposed to hang out. But you seem nice, so we thought you probably wouldn't tell on us!"

"Err … No, of course not. But I didn't realise we weren't allowed to socialise …"

"I know, it's a crap rule, isn't it?" Rachel butts in. "I wonder what they'd do if they found out!"

"So do all of you go out together then?"

"Except for Caroline. She's ... different. I mean, don't get me wrong, she's lovely and everything; but I don't know if she'd approve." I wonder what made them think I was 'nice' and different from Caroline, but I feel quite flattered. We go to a place called The King's Head, not far from the Hospital. As I don't want to get drunk in front of them, I order an Archers and Lemonade - I was going to get an orange juice, but as they all bought beer, I thought they might find me boring.

"So what do you think of the therapy so far?" Renee asks. I feel awfully self-conscious and worried I might say the wrong thing. What if they all think it's the best thing they've ever come across?

"Err ... It's still early days ..."

"Don't you find Chrissie really annoying?" Rachel asks and the other two nod.

"Well, actually, kind of, yes."

"I think this is much more helpful than any therapy!"

"Definitely. She's so patronising. Who's your individual therapist?"

"John. He doesn't say much."

"No, he doesn't. Sometimes he stares at me in silence; the first time he did that he really freaked me out!" Rachel says, laughing.

"I think he's trying to get to know you; he did that with me at first. Now he interacts with me more." Adam says, breaking off his long silence at last.

"But I've been in therapy for months!" Rachel answers.

"I was talking to Melanie. Maybe he's just not interested in you." Adam says with a grin. I get the feeling I'm not the only one who finds Rachel annoying. But she doesn't seem to take the hint.

"He's not supposed to be interested in me, he's supposed to help me!"

"Where do you work, Melanie?" Adam asks as though he hadn't heard her.

"I'm in Market Research. It's not very interesting. What about you?" I hope I don't have anything stuck in my teeth.

"Adam is a lady of leisure!" Rachel says in a giggle.

"I don't work, thank you Rachel."

"How come?"

"I don't like the idea. I want to be a writer, so I write; but I haven't been published yet."

"But … how do you manage to pay for things?"

"I'm on benefits."

"Really?" I've never met anyone on benefits before.

"And that gives you enough to live on?"

"Not exactly. My parents help."

"That's … very nice of them."

"Isn't he a lucky sod? Your taxes pay for his rent!"

"Huh … But … don't you have to be looking for work to be on benefits?"

"If you're on the dole, yeah. I'm on Incapacity Benefits."

"It's the crazy people's benefits!" Rachel shouts again. He frowns.

"So you're actually unfit to work?"

"I am unstable, yeah."

"So are we, but we still have jobs!" Renee says finally. They both seem fairly cross with Adam. I suppose it's understandable; I mean, apparently, I have issues, and I manage to work. In a way, I'm working to pay for his rent and food and everything else. That seems wrong.

"I know I'm lucky. I get to do what I want, which is writing. You three are working, and none of you seem to enjoy it. But that's not my fault."

"So what do you write about?" I ask in an awkward attempt to change the subject.

"My life, more or less."

"Your life? Is it that interesting?" Somehow that didn't sound as bad in my head. He seems quite offended. Shit. "What I meant was …"

"No, you're right, he's a pretentious bastard!" Rachel interrupts again. I wonder if being in therapy would give me a good enough excuse to commit murder.

"I didn't mean it like that …" I say again, trying to look at him, but my eyes can't reach higher than his nose. I think I'm blushing.

"That's OK." He smiles, and I get the strange feeling that I'm going to melt.

****

I wonder if he has a girlfriend. He hasn't mentioned one yet. But then, he never says much in sessions. He must have, he's too good looking not too. And even if he didn't, what chance do I have? He's probably into tall busty blondes. Maybe he's gay. Maybe James could tell. But what if I introduce him to James and he doesn't like him and thinks I have crap friends? And maybe he's not straight but he's not gay either yet and James will convert him! I can't risk that. But how can I find out? If I ask Renee or Rachel they'll think I'm after him. And I'm not. Not yet. I'm … not sure. I do like him. He seems different. The rare times that I talk in the group, he always says 'I agree', or 'I feel the same way', when Chrissie asks him what he thinks. And he wouldn't say that if he didn't mean it, would he? There's no point thinking about it anyway. I'm not going there again. Not after what happened with Simon. Maybe he's a rapist or a serial killer! What do I know? He's in therapy, isn't he? And why would he like me more than Renee? She's nice. I'm sure every guy fancies her. He's so lucky to do what he wants. I don't know what I'd do if I weren't in Market Research, but I know at this stage I'd rather do pretty much anything else. Well, maybe not anything; I wouldn't want to be a doctor, especially not a gynaecologist; nor a rubbish collector. I wonder what Adam's books are like. I'd love to read them. He must have had a really interesting life, to write about it. My life story would fit into one chapter.

"Mel? I've got some weirdo on the phone and I can't understand what she's saying", a new girl called Abigail says, interrupting my thinking.

"Why can't you understand her? Is she foreign?"

"No, but she's disabled or something. She keeps stuttering and making funny noises!" She giggles, looking at a guy next to her and he laughs as well. She's only been here a week and she already thinks she runs the place.

"But is she answering the questions?"

"Yeah. But…"

"If she answers the questions you need to finish the interview", I say as calmly as I can.

"But I could have done at least five interviews for all the time I've wasted with her. Can't I just put the phone down?"

"Why would you do that?"

"Well … What's the point of talking to her?"

"So because she's disabled her opinion doesn't count? Is that what you're saying?" I can't help picturing the people at Mary's. Everyone is looking at me now, but I don't care. How dare she? Now she's just sitting there in silence. I bet she wasn't expecting me to tell her off. I bet no one did. They thought I'd just let her take the piss out of me.

"Just put them through to Melanie. She'll finish the interview" I hear Philip say behind me. I don't believe it. How could he do this to me?

"I don't understand." I say to him after the end of the shift. "Surely you knew she was in the wrong!"

"I did. And that's why I let you deal with it. She wasn't taking the person seriously, and I don't think the interview would have been worth a lot if she'd finished it herself. Was the lady incoherent?"

"She spoke slowly and babbled a lot, but I understood her."

"Exactly. Because you're experienced. And, from what I know, you have come across people with mental disabilities. Abigail obviously hasn't."

"But you embarrassed me in front of the whole team! How are they going to take me seriously now?"

"They will, and they already do, believe me. They know how good you are. Melanie, do you realise that only a few weeks ago, you wouldn't have dared to come into my office and tell me how you felt? You've gained a lot of confidence.

"Oh" is all I can manage. I don't know what to make of that. In a way, it's nice that he thinks I'm confident, but how do I know that's a good thing to him? Maybe he only likes people when they kiss his arse. And 'a few weeks ago', I wouldn't have felt any worse than I just did, in front of everyone.

****

"I wonder what makes you feel this way", John says in his usual reflective tone, in my session the next day.

"What way?"

"Well … You quite often mention thoughts of others disliking you, talking about you behind your back and even humiliating you. I wonder what triggers that."

"What triggers people not to like me? I don't know! Because they're crap? Because I'm crap? Ask them!"

"I didn't mean what triggers people not to like you, but what triggers you to think that they don't."

"You've lost me. Surely that's the same thing."

"I don't think it is. I don't think asking you where you bought a top from because it looks nice is a sign that someone dislikes you. Or showing concern about your eating and drinking. I wonder if maybe it is easier for you to think that people are against you, than that they are your friends."

"How is that easier? Do you think I enjoy being left out? Do you think I like being a laughing stock?"

"I didn't say that you enjoyed it. But maybe you are more scared of people liking you, because you're scared of becoming too attached to them and then lose them. That could be why you have rejected the idea of having a relationship."

"I don't understand how you can make this kind of assumption when you've only known me five minutes."

"I'm only saying this based on what you told me. Maybe you need some time to reflect on it. We do have to finish now." This is what he does every time. He says something that really upsets me, then tells me to 'reflect on it', making it clear I have to shut up until next time. And who do I talk to until then ? I haven't said anything to James. He's far too happy to understand. Maybe I could speak to Adam. Or Renee. But they've got their own problems, they don't need mine. It would be nice, though. I've got their numbers … No. That would just be silly. It's not like they care anyway. I need a drink. And some food. Lots of it. No! I can't. I have to be strong. I can't put on weight. Adam would hate me then. Maybe I should do something sporty. But what ? I can't go to the gym because I'm not registered ; I can't run because I'm on my own and I'd be too embarrassed ; and I can't swim either; there's no way I'm letting anyone see me half naked. It's fate, telling me I shouldn't bother trying to make an effort. I was born fat and ugly and I shall remain it. So I may as well get fatter and uglier.

I stop at Sainsbury's on the way back. I haven't been paid yet, so I can't afford much. And I hate carrying lots of bags anyway. I start with the wine section; I want to put off looking at food for as long as I can.

" Having a party ?" I turn around, only to see Adam stand in front of me!

" Oh. Hi !" I can't believe it. I'm so glad I don't have any food in my basket! " Err … No, I just … err … "

"Fancied a drink ? Me too. I'm having beer though. I hate wine." I try not to look at him. He's so handsome. He always wears these long sleeves jumpers, like a philosophy student or something. He must be a bit hot, though.

" I didn't know you live around here ?" I proudly manage to say without babbling.

" I don't. But there's a music shop I really like in Wood Green, so I come here sometimes. And I felt like having a drink on the way back."

" What did you get ?" I ask pointing at his bag.

" Some bands you've probably never heard of." I'm quite offended by that. How does he know ? He obviously thinks I'm boring.

" I might know them", I say trying not to sound too defensive.

" Vega 4, Black Car and Arch Enemy."

" Err … No. I've never heard of them." As he smiles, I'm blushing.

" So what do you like?" If I tell him he'll never speak to him again.

" You know … This and that. I have varied tastes."

" Me too. Apart from rap and pop."

"Me too!" I say way too enthusiastically and he laughs. Crap.

"Good."

"Yes." I don't know what to do now. Is he expecting me to say something else, ask him questions? "So … What are you up to now?"

"Well, I've finished my shopping, so I was just going to go home and arse around. You?"

"The same, probably."

"Do you fancy arsing around together then?" Oh God! I do, but I don't as well. What if I say something stupid and he doesn't want to see me ever again? Or if I'm not intelligent enough?

"Err …"

"You don't have to."

"No! I want to. I mean, yes, OK!"

We buy a few drinks; wine, beer and some plastic cups (I don't want him to see me drink wine out of the bottle). We take a bus to Hampstead Heath and sit in the park. He suggested we had a picnic, but there's no way I'm eating in front of him. We sit on the grass, in front of a pond. There's hardly anyone around; just birds, ducks and squirrels. I should have brought some nuts or bread to give them. We talk for hours and even the simplest things he says seem so meaningful. I tell him about the hospital … and he's really supportive. He says he admires the way I handled it and that I'm very strong. Night falls too quickly … I don't want to leave. Thankfully, we arrange to meet again at the weekend. He says he has a few places in mind that I might like. He insists on taking me all the way back to my house and for a moment I think he might want to come in; but he just gives me a hug and goes away. Which is nice, in a way … but I guess we're just friends. How many men will walk you back home without expecting something else? I feel pathetic for letting myself fall for it. What chance did I have?

"He sounds perfect!" James says after I tell him about it. "He obviously likes you."

"What makes you think that? If you're interested in someone, you shag them straight away, don't you?"

"Yeah, but not all men are tarts, believe it or not. He probably didn't want to rush things."

"Or he just doesn't fancy me."

"Don't be stupid. Everyone fancies you!"

"Yeah, right."

"Of course they do! Even women! The two over there, they haven't stopped staring at you."

"How do you know that they're gay anyway?"

"Honey. We're in a gay pub. And they make Vin Diesel look like a ballerina." It does seem like they're looking at me, but I doubt it's in the way James thinks. They're making fun of me, more like. They keep smiling and whispering to each other. I wonder what it is this time. My t-shirt? My hair? My lack of makeup?

"Oi!"

"What?"

"I thought I'd lost you. What were you thinking about? You seemed miles away."

"Nothing really. What should I do about Adam? I'm scared I'll get drunk next time and make a fool of myself."

"You worry too much. Just take it easy with him. He's probably as nervous as you are." I think James understands straight men even less than I do. What has he got to be nervous about?

"How did you meet him again?" Damn. I didn't think about that.

"Err … through work."

"Work? But I thought you said he didn't work?"

"Oh. No, he doesn't. Well, he did, just for a day. He didn't like it."

"And you kept in touch after knowing him for only a day?"

"Yeah. Why is that so strange?"

"No reason. He must be a hell of a hunk though. I just thought it'd take you at least a year to decide if you like someone."

"Only took me a couple of days with you though, didn't it?"

"Yes, but that's different."

"And why's that?"

"Because I'm lovely."

"Well so is he!"

"So did he ask for your number?" I'm offended by this.

"No, actually. I did." OK. Highly unlikely, but so what?

"Really? Good for you! Anyway, I'm starving. Wanna get some food? I fancy something nice." Oh no. I'm too stressed to eat. If I start now, I won't stop.

"I'm OK. But I'll come with you." James's idea of 'nice food' is a chicken burger and extra large fries at McDonald's. I hate fast food places. Just the smell of them makes me put on weight.

"I got you something." He hands me a tray with things similar to his.

"What's all this?"

"I didn't believe you weren't hungry. And even if you're not, one bite of this and you'll be grateful!" I can't believe he did that. Is he trying to torture me?

"James! I told you I didn't want anything!" I cry, shaking.

"Sorry. I didn't realise it'd put you in such a state. I'll just bin it." He rolls his eyes and sighs.

"Don't worry. I'll eat some." But obviously, I don't just eat 'some', I eat the whole damn thing. Every bite I take is agony, but I can't help it. I don't want it, I certainly don't need it, but I have to have it.

"See? I knew you were hungry!" I feel sick and guilty for betraying my body once again.

"I've got to go to the loo." I get up and look around for the toilets. That's another thing I hate about McDonald's; they're always dirty and there's usually only one or two cubicles. As I wait for my turn, a queue forms behind me. Great. It'll be impossible to do anything here. Shit! I can't get any fatter, I just can't! I know what'll happen if I throw up here. People will hear, they'll make a fuss about it and everyone will know, including James.

"I have to go home", I say when I come back.

"But it's only eight!"

"Sorry. I just don't feel well. It must have been that burger."

"That's because your body's not used to food. Look at yourself! If I didn't know you, I'd say you're an anorexic." The word hits me harder than any slap I've ever received. I'm not anorexic! I just don't like food! It's like an allergy. And anyway, I'm too fat to be anorexic! Even John's never used that word before.

"Don't be stupid! I'm just not bothered about food, that's all."

"You seemed bothered a minute ago when I tried to give you some." The looks he gives me could mean, 'I'm worried', or 'you're insane'. I feel like I'm dealing with Naomi again. I don't want us to end up like me and her.

"Look, I'm not anorexic, honestly. I'm just not too keen on fast food. I'm even considering becoming vegetarian."

"Really? Why?"

"It's … healthier."

"Less fattening, you mean." Is he a bloody mind reader?

I was hoping he'd call some friends and stay out, but instead, he wants to go home as well, which means I probably won't be able to be sick there either. I wish I didn't have to share the toilets. But then, it occurs to me that, actually, if he did hear me, he'd know I wasn't lying when I said I wasn't feeling well. So I do and as his room is next to the toilets, it's not long before he comes out and knocks on the door.

"Mel? Is that you? Are you OK?"

"I'll be fine … Must have been the burger."

****

Nothing to wear. I have absolutely nothing to wear. What am I going to do? I can't go out looking like a tramp, can I? I've only got three hours and I haven't even started my makeup. Yes, I intend to put on makeup. I don't have a choice! This was a mistake, I should never have agreed to meet him. I'll bore him to death and soon enough he'll be chatting up some girls and I'll look even more stupid. I should just stay home with my wine and a film. I'm really tempted to cancel. But then I'll never be able to show my face at the group again. Why does everything I own make me look even fatter! I did ask James for advice - being gay, I thought he'd know about these things, he said he'd give me a hand, but now he's nowhere to be seen. The only thing that vaguely fits is a long black skirt and a quarter length shirt. As I know even less about makeup than about men and don't actually own much of it, all I can do is put on a bit of eyeliner, some greyish eye shadow and mulled wine lipstick – as carefully chosen by Naomi on one of our, then, inflicted monthly trips to Brent Cross shopping centre. I drink some wine to calm my nerves, but when I finally drag myself out of the flat, I'm shaking like a leaf. I walk to the tube station and on the way a couple of men whistle as I walk past them. I don't understand; do they expect me to turn around and talk to them? Thank you for treating me like a piece of meat, would you like a drink? I bet if I did that, they'd run off like thieves. I hate the tube. It's so hot, packed with scruffy people who'd push you on the rails just to get on a train. And the stares I get – I'm sitting in front of a large man with round glasses and a beard and he's been eying me since I sat down. It's Friday night and everyone's out, holding cans of beer or doing their makeup. Another man grins as I meet his eyes; even a teenager! Why? Why me? You don't need to remind me that I'm ugly! You don't need to make fun of me! I can't do this. I knew it was a bad idea. Who am I kidding? He'll never want me.

Leicester Square. That's where we're supposed to meet. But I won't come out of the station. I'll just get off the train and catch one back to Turnpike Lane. I'll get a video and some more wine, and I'll go home. I'll switch my phone off so …

"Melanie!" It's Adam. Christ, is he stalking me? I could run off, or tell him I'm ill or something. But I don't.

"Hi."

"Hi. We must have been on the same train, I guess." We go to a bar near the station, where the furniture seems out of an Austin Powers film and the music is an interesting and somewhat unusual mix of jazz and disco. The drinks are expensive, but he insists on buying most of them. As always, he hardly looks at me and it makes me wonder if he'd rather be with anyone else here. But he talks, a lot, only pausing to take a sip of his beer or when he expects a comment from me. I'm happy to let him talk; he's so interesting. He's travelled the world, mixed with the rich and poor, the good and the evil. His last girlfriend was a kleptomaniac.

"I came back from Holland after two weeks backpacking; she hadn't come because she hadn't renewed her passport on time. She'd practically emptied my flat and let my dog starve to death."

"That's awful. Did you go to the police?"

"Yeah. But they had no proof she'd done it. She denied that she was ever asked to look after the dog. After that, I didn't go out for a month. My mum had to bring me food. I couldn't even see my friends. I didn't trust anyone." I try hard to think of something equally sad and dramatic to say about myself, but I can't. He must think I'm pathetic, complaining about my life when he's obviously had it far worse. "Anyway, there's this club I think you'd like. We could have a couple of drinks in another bar, and go there afterwards."

"A Club? Great!" The idea gives me stomach cramps. I haven't been to a club for years! I can't dance! I'm going to embarrass myself so much. "So … What kind of club are we going to?" I ask, trying not to sound terrified.

"It's a place not far. The music's quite varied and the drinks aren't too dear."

"Good." With a bit of luck, by the time we get there we'll both be too drunk to move a toe. I wonder if he's having a good time. Maybe he wants to go to a club because he's bored of talking to me! I loathe Central London, especially on Friday night. Everyone shouting and drinking on the streets, it's so primitive.

"Are you OK?" He asks as we get into a pub called The George.

"Yes! Why?"

"No reason. Have you ever had absinthe?"

"No. Isn't it illegal?"

"Not anymore. Want to try some?"

"Err … Sure." I insist on buying the round and I'm given a shot glass containing a bright green liquid.

"It's really strong. You have to drink it in one go."

"Right." I've never seen the point in wasting money on a drink I won't have time to taste, but I don't want to sound moaney or tight.

"And don't smell it! Ready?" I swallow and choke. I've never drunk anything so vile. It's perfume! "Strong, isn't it?"

"I … don't think I'll be having another one!" My throat feels like it's on fire; after a few seconds of heavy coughing, though, my head suddenly begins to lighten and the rest of my body follows soon after. I close my eyes and imagine being on a boat, floating on a quiet sea. I've no idea what music is playing, or who's around me; I'm in a parallel dimension and it's just me and the elements. Five, ten minutes or maybe an hour pass, I've completely lost sense of time and rationality. When I open my eyes again, I'm in his arms and he stares at me with a big smile.

So I grab his head, move it towards mine and kiss him. It's only later on that I realise how embarrassing it would have been if he'd turned me down … but he doesn't. And when I ask him if I can spend the night with him, he says yes straight away. We catch the last train to his house – my place is far too messy – have some more drinks, talk, and kiss more. A lot more. And all I can think of is whether he wants me and how much. I soon find out, when he slowly undoes my top; too slowly for my liking.

"You can tell I haven't done this for a while!" I hear him say. So I help him. Usually, I would have been too nervous to move a muscle, but the alcohol has made me feel more confident than ever. It's as though, all of a sudden, I'd turned into a gorgeous, fearless vixen. And when I wake up in the morning, although confused at first and badly hung-over, I'm the happiest I've been in years. I can't believe it's happened. I can't believe I'm with him! I pinch myself to make sure I'm not dreaming, but it's all real! I bet my makeup is all over, though. And my bag is miles away and if I get up I'll probably wake him up and then I'll have to look at him! Thankfully, there's a mirror on his bedside table. I lean over him as gently as I can to reach it, and that's when my so newly found perfect world falls apart: here is, in front of me, the reason why Adam always wears jumpers. Since I haven't noticed any tigers in his flat, I conclude that the dozens of cuts and scars on his arms were self-inflicted. Adam self-harms. He cuts himself. He takes a knife, a razor blade, maybe even scissors, and makes his skin bleed. I'm so shocked. I stare at his arms, unable to move. Why didn't he say anything? Did he think I wouldn't notice?

"Hey." I look away, not saying anything. "Everything OK?"

"I don't know. Is it?"

"Did I snore? I'm sorry if I did, I'm not usually ..."

"You didn't snore."

"What then? Do you ... regret what happened last night?"

"No. I don't know. It's just ... why didn't you tell me about your cuts?" He looks down and stays silent for a moment.

"Oh."

"Did you think I wouldn't see them?"

"Well ... yeah. I was drunk; I guess I forgot to cover them."

"But why not telling me?"

"Because I wanted to avoid this kind of reaction. Look, I'm sorry. I just … didn't want you to freak out."

"So you lied to me? You lied to me to get me into bed!"

"I didn't lie to you. I was worried that you'd reject me."

"Why did you never say anything in the group?"

"Because I don't want people to know. It's not something I'm proud of", he says in a shaky voice. His expression is similar to my sister's when I used to tell her off.

"I'm sorry. I'm just … in shock. I wasn't expecting to see that. It looks really … painful."

"I'm immune to the pain now. I have to cut really deep to feel anything these days." Just the thought of it makes me cringe.

"Is that why you do it? To feel pain?"

"Sort of. I do it because I'm hurting mentally; the physical pain makes me forget about what's in my head for a while."

"What goes on in your head that makes you want to do this?" I point at his arms, trying not to look disgusted.

"It's not a nice place to be. It's like a big room full of stuff, but nowhere to put it all. No drawers, no cupboard, it's all spread out on the floor. A mess. That's what it is."

"I'd never thought about it that way. I guess it's quite similar to my situation."

"But you don't cut?"

"No." I couldn't deal with the scars. It was bad enough when I did it in the park; I couldn't go through that on a regular basis.

"How do you cope then?"

"I don't. I just get angry at myself and everyone else; I'm miserable. I drink. I get sick."

"What do you mean, get sick?" Since he's told me his secret, I might as well tell him mine.

"I make myself sick."

"No wonder you're so skinny. How often do you do it?"

"I don't know ... I don't really want to talk about it."

"And I didn't really want to discuss my arms, but we've been on the subject for a few minutes now." I guess he's right.

"I haven't counted. I just do it when I feel like it."

"That's another form of self harm, you know. You're hurting your body as much as I am, if not more. You're causing permanent damage to your liver."

"Maybe, but that's my problem. At least my scars are internal."

"They're the worst."

"I don't think so! Are you planning to wear long sleeves for the rest of your life?"

"It's like you said. It's my problem." I want to say, actually, it's mine too now, but I don't know if it is. He hasn't said anything about getting together. Maybe he just wanted sex. And that's just as well. I don't think I could deal with his issues.

"I should go."

"What?"

"I said I should go."

"So that's it?"

"Well ... Isn't that what you want?"

"You spend one night with me and you think you know me? You think you know what I want?"

"I just thought …"

"Forget it. You're just like everyone else. Go away." His face has turned red and his whole body seems really tense. For the first time since I've met him I feel scared. "Why are you still here? Get the fuck out of my flat!" So I do. I run off and swear never to return. How could he? And how could I give myself to such a psycho? I should have known there'd be something wrong with him. It was just too good to be true. I let him touch me, use me, only to insult and humiliate me! He thinks he's so cool because he's written a couple of books and goes to the gym, but guess what? You're so not! A fucking loser and a waste of space, that's what you are! And a self harming freak!

****

Needless to say I don't attend Monday's group session. It's not that I'm embarrassed or anything, but I'm making a point and this point is that I don't want to see his pasty face ever again. I was hoping for a call or a text from Renee or Rachel to see if I was OK, but no one bothered. He must have told them what happened and they're obviously on his side. Or maybe they don't know but just don't give a toss what happens to me. I can't even tell John about it; for all I know Adam might mention it to him as well and then he'll put two and two together and I'll get into trouble. Maybe they'll throw me out of the programme. Not that it's done me any good so far, but it's the only thing I can hold on to. John finds me "gloomy, downbeat and darker than usual". He asks questions, what triggered it, last week I seemed so hyper and excited, almost radiant. But I manage not to give away anything. And then, he says it. The one thing I was hoping never to hear again after seeing that doctor in Lordship. "Anti depressants. I think it's an option worth considering."

"I'd rather not. I don't see the point." But despite that, he gives me a prescription.

"Think about it. If you really don't want to, just throw it away. But at least give it a think first." So I have it. The proof that I'm now officially mad. I'm holding it in my hand. A tiny white pill. In it, I'm supposed to find what nothing else could give me. The world will be a great place, people will become human and I will love it all. It might as well say that on the packet, because that's what I'd want to take it for. Not for the nausea, the diarrhoea, the irritations and dozens of other side effects stated on the box – and certainly not for the suicidal thoughts. If you want to get better, take anti depressants; but before you notice any improvement, be prepared to feel shit. Really, really badly. In fact, you might end up killing yourself. But we thank you for giving us your money. So I stare at it, wondering if it is the one thing that's been missing; the solution to my problems. But are they addictive? Could I spend my life on drugs? John said you usually only stay on them for six months or a year, maybe two in extreme cases. But there could be exceptions, I'm sure. I mean, Americans are all hooked on them. He also said that it takes at least a few weeks before they start working, but the side effects kick in after just three or four days. So if I get headaches, dry mouth or even panic attacks, I should just "bide my time". Citalopram, that's what my drug is called. It's like Prozac, apparently. I couldn't tell the difference anyway. I'm still not sure about this. If I take it, there'll be no turning back. Even if I only have the one, I'll spend the rest of my life knowing that once, I was on Prozac. I wish someone was here to hold my hand. It's as though I were about to make a big jump and there's no one to catch me. Adam could catch me. He's strong enough. But he hasn't even tried to apologise. It's been nearly two weeks and I've heard nothing. Maybe he's dead. He cut too deep and reached a vein. I shouldn't care, really. It's not like I did anything wrong. But I do care. I still like him. Don't ask me why. But he's not here. It's just me and a little pill. My new ally, maybe. My life jacket.

****

    I don't notice any changes in the first few days. I go to a couple of bars with James on Saturday, but as I'm not supposed to drink whilst on the tablets (I don't intend to stick to that rule for long), the evening is pretty dull. But come Tuesday and I'm woken up by the most horrific headache. I drag myself to work but can't face going to therapy. When I get back home I go straight to bed, but after two hours of tossing and turning, I decide to run a bath. As I come out of my room the doorbell goes. I never usually answer it, but whoever's outside is more than likely to have seen me as the front door is partly made of smoked glass, so I open it and jump. It's Adam.

"What ... What are you doing here?"

"I just wanted to check if you were alright. You weren't at the group."

"I had a headache. I'm fine. Now, if you'll excuse me, I'm going to take a bath."

"Can we talk?"

"About what?"

"Us."

"There's no us."

"Look, I'm sorry about what happened. I didn't mean to upset you."

"Whatever. I have to go now."

"Can't you give me a chance to explain?"

"You've had almost two weeks. It's a bit late now, don't you think? And anyway, I … Hang on. How did you know where I live?"

"I followed you after your session on Thursday." Oh my God.

"You followed me?"

"I needed to know that you were OK. That you were … still alive."

"You didn't have to follow me all the way to my house to see that!" I'm struggling not to shake, but I'm really starting to feel scared again.

"I wanted to talk to you, but I couldn't do it on the street. That's why I followed you here. But then, I couldn't bring myself to do it."

"Are you stalking me?"

"Of course not! I just really needed to see you. Please, let me in. Give me five minutes." So I do, not so much because I want to, but rather for fear of his reaction if I closed the door on him. After over an hour of apologies and begging for forgiveness, I give in and we end up in bed.

"Melanie, I would never hurt you", he says as he undoes my bra. "You're so special."

It feels strange to have sex completely sober, so I let him take control. By the time we're done, my headache is long forgotten.

Chapter 6

So that's my vow of celibacy out of the window. It's really strange, actually. Not long ago I thought I wouldn't be with anyone ever again. I kind of feel like a hypocrite. But it's all happening so quickly! Thing is, since I've never been in love, I don't know what it's like to feel it. I'm very fond of him; but how could I tell if it's love or just the excitement of being with someone? He treats me well, he's kind, affectionate and very intelligent. I wouldn't be with him if he weren't all that. But now that I've found someone, it makes me wonder if maybe there's an even better person out there. I don't believe in soul mates. Sure, some people click, but they can't be completely similar; or if they were, they'd get bored of each other very quickly. I think he likes me more than I like him. I told him we should only see each other three or four times a week and he seemed quite disappointed. But I can't spend all my time with him, I need my own space. I don't see why he'd want to see me any more though, it's not like I have anything interesting to talk about. Maybe he needs the company.

He mentions his friends a lot, but so far I've only met a couple of them. They're both nice enough, I suppose. One is a wannabe filmmaker, the other works at the Tate, so apparently we could get in for free. I'm not too keen on art though, but I haven't told Adam. Renee and Rachel don't know about us yet; it's been over a month since the first time we slept together, but we just don't know how to break it to them. I bet they'll be jealous of me, because it's obvious they fancy him. Everyone does. I actually can't quite believe he chose me when he could have the most gorgeous girls in the world! I'd love to know what he sees in me. But I won't ask him yet in case it makes him think about it too much. Whenever we meet, I half expect him to end it, but we always find ourselves in bed. I don't really enjoy it though; not that he's not good or gentle or anything, but I'm always so tense and worried that I'm not up to his standards. We never do it with the light on; I refuse to let him see me naked. At first, he thought it was because of his scars. He got really upset, so I had to tell him the truth. Of course he said I was mad, I shouldn't worry about anything because I'm so skinny, all the usual. The other thing is, we've started going out at the wrong time. It's November and that means my birthday's just around the corner. I hate birthdays. At school, I was never invited to parties; once, my mother organised one for me and the only person who turned up was my neighbour and she didn't even have a kid. I spent the day crying in bed and made my mother swear never to do it again. Of course once I met Naomi, we spent our birthdays together. We usually went to the cinema and had cake (or usually fruit salad, in my case) in the local coffee shop. This year, I'll pretend I don't have one. I hate being the centre of attention and I would hate to think that he felt obliged to buy me something. So I shall spend the day by myself.

My mother doesn't know I don't speak to Naomi anymore, so she thinks we'll be doing the usual. And I haven't told her about Adam either. I don't want them to meet. She would no doubt embarrass me and he'd probably scare her off and that would be another excuse for her to criticise me. She's only ever met one of my boyfriends. She thinks I'm gay. She's never said it directly, but there have been many innuendos. I thought I was at one stage … Or rather, I'd decided to be gay. I was convinced that women were nicer and less interested in looks than men; when I was seventeen, I went to a lesbian club and I was sure that my long hair and nail polish would make me stand out and I'd pull easily. But the people who did notice me had looks on their face that seemed to say "you don't belong here" more than "I want to shag you." I spent the whole night drinking by myself at the bar. So I realised women were just as bad. James thought it was hilarious; he thinks I'd "make a great lesbian", and offered to introduce me to a couple of his girlfriends; but I nicely told him that I wouldn't know what to do with one, since I can't even give myself an orgasm.

I always get a card from work on my birthday. I don't have to remind them, not that I would anyway. Phil keeps a diary of everyone's "big day", as he puts it. Thankfully, no one earns enough to buy presents, so I'm always spared the tacky ornaments and book vouchers. I still have to act pleased and thank everyone for writing the same meaningless crap every year.

"I've made breakfast." Adam comes in holding a tray with two cups, orange juice and about half a loaf worth of toast.

"Thanks. I'll just have the coffee."

"And toast? There's jam and margarine."

"You know I don't eat in the morning."
"Well, it's time you did. No wonder you're always tired."

"I'm always tired?" Or does he mean I always look like shit?

"That's what you say. It doesn't surprise me. Your body needs carbs in the morning."

"My body needs caffeine. You didn't put sugar in that, did you?" He sighs.

"No. So, when can I see you again?"

"I don't know. Next week?"

"Have you got any plans?"

"Don't think so."

"Good. The Sound of Music is on and I thought you might want to see it. I could come over with some drinks."

"I love The Sound of Music! When is it?"

"Tuesday." Damn. That's my birthday.

"Oh."

"Is that a problem?"

"No. It's just … Nothing. That's fine."

"Great." He drinks his coffee, has a shower and leaves for his session with John. On Tuesday, I get the birthday call from my mother, a text from Jenny and of course, a card from work. I watch The Sound of Music with Adam, get drunk and fall asleep in his arms. The next morning however, isn't so great. When I wake up, I find him sitting on the bed, staring at me, the birthday card in his hand. I'd thrown it away before he got here yesterday.

"What's this?" He asks in a shaky voice.

"A card."

"I can see that. Why didn't you tell me it was your birthday?"

"Sorry, but why exactly were you going through my bin?"

"I was clearing up the mess we'd left yesterday."

"Why? Did you think I couldn't manage?"

"I was trying to be nice! Anyway, I asked you a question."

"I didn't want it to be a big deal."

"A big deal? Don't you think sooner or later I was going to ask you when your birthday was?"

"I … don't know. I would have made up a date."

"Made up a date?" He repeats, like an angry parrot. "And you don't think that's making it a bigger deal than it actually is?"

"I'm just not used to people being nice to me. It … scares me."

"But why? I'm your boyfriend. It's my job to be nice to you!" Then I cry and he cries and begs me to let him take me to dinner that evening. He picks me up from work and for a little while I'm the most popular person in the office. "Is that your bloke? He's gorgeous!" He takes me to an Italian, we both order salads and just before settling the bill, he hands me a little box wrapped in purple paper. Inside is the most beautiful bracelet I've ever seen.

"You shouldn't have. It's beautiful."
"Really? You like it?"

"I love it", I say, my eyes watering. It's too much kindness for one evening.

****

I now get an idea of what it's like to be pregnant. Thanks to these stupid pills, I wake up every morning with nausea and throwing up doesn't seem to make it any better. I don't know how long I can handle this for. Not only that and the headaches, but now my face is covered in small spots and I had to cancel seeing Adam because I was too embarrassed. I'm beginning to miss him when he's not around, especially at night. It's nice to snuggle up with him. The first few times, I didn't get any sleep for fear of snoring or dribbling, but I'm getting better. He sleeps so heavily that I don't think anything would wake him up. He used to wear long sleeves in bed, but I told him not to. I don't want him to be embarrassed. But the truth is, I hate looking at his arms.

I don't understand how a razor blade can make you forget about your problems. I don't see the need to carve "evil" on your shoulder. Thankfully, I don't think he's done it since we've got together, but I know it'll happen sooner or later. Probably next time we argue. Apparently, after I stormed out of his flat, he cut for over three hours. I couldn't believe the state of him when he showed me. I felt quite guilty of course, but also flattered that I could have caused him so much pain. He wants me to meet his parents. Apparently he's told them all about me, so now I bet they're shitting themselves. And so am I. I don't want them to dislike me. I only met one of my exes' mothers and it didn't matter to me what she thought because I knew I wouldn't stay with him for long. I'm kind of hoping it'll last with Adam. Maybe I can make him stop the cutting.

"I think we should tell them", he declares one day out of the blue. "It's been a while now."

"Do we have to?"

"I'm tired of sitting opposite you every time we're with them. I'm tired of pretending I don't know you. I've nothing to hide."

"Well, actually ..." I say looking at his arms.

"You know what I mean."

"Fine. If you really want to. But I don't think it'll go down well."

"Why not? I think they'll be pleased."

"Pleased?" I can't help giggling. "What would they have to be pleased about?"

"That two of their friends have got together?" I shake my head and sigh, not saying any more. I wish he weren't so naive. Of course they're not "happy", they don't welcome us with open arms and there's no "congratulations". "Oh", is what we get.

"When did this happen?"

"About a month ago", Adam says, staring at his empty pint.

"A month ago? And you waited until now to tell us?"

"I know it seems like a long time," he continues, "but we weren't sure how to bring it up".

"So all this time you guys pretended to be friends. You were playing with us!"

"It wasn't like that."

"You're very quiet" Rachel says, looking at me accusingly. I look down, pinching my leg so I don't lose my temper.

"I ... don't know what to say."

"You could tell us how it happened", she says still staring at me, her arms crossed. So I tell them the story that we agreed on: I bumped into him in a club, we were both drunk and next thing I know it's Saturday morning and I'm in his bed. But they don't look any less angry.

"Are you going to tell Chrissie?" I let Adam answer once again.

"I don't know. It wouldn't go down well."

"You have to tell her. You can't go on like this forever. It's not doing either of you any favour and it's not fair on us."

"But what if she throws us out?" I cry.

"Well, you should have thought of that before throwing yourself at him!" Rachel shouts. I knew she'd be jealous.

"I'm sure they wouldn't throw you out", Renee says at last. "But I agree with Rachel, you should tell her. What will happen the day you have an argument and want to talk about it in the group? Or you want to say something without the other one knowing about it? You can hardly do that if you're sitting next to each other." She's right. Of course she is.

"But we never talk anyway!" I hear Adam say, half laughing. "Even before we started going out, it's always been about you!" He adds, pointing at Rachel.

"Well then, I don't see why you're so worried about getting thrown out!"

I leave Adam to deal with them soon after. He wanted to follow me, but I insisted he stayed. I need time on my own. I'm angry at him for not listening to me and thinking he knew better. Actually, I'm rather furious. I hope they have a right go at him. I hope they make him feel stupid. But what if they don't? What if, instead, they make him feel that it's my entire fault and talk him into dumping me? What if Rachel comes onto him? And how come I left over an hour ago and he hasn't rung me yet?

I feel like shit. This is undoubtedly the worst I've felt since I started talking those flaming pills. I don't even have the energy to get out of bed. I called in sick. Couldn't face work. Couldn't face the operators' fake happy voices, the angry customers complaining about their interviews, couldn't face the mess in the kitchen, the noise, Philip, James, the bus, I just couldn't. I haven't told Adam, because I know he'd want to come over if I did. Couldn't see him either. I thought being with him would change me. I thought I'd be normal. But I'm still how I was before. Occasionally, I feel slightly more positive; but that scares me even more than depression. At least, I'm used to depression. I know what it is and what it does to me. But happiness is an obscure notion, something I've never been properly introduced to and so when it's there, I don't know what to do with it. Why bother being happy anyway? It'll all blow up in your face in the end. Sooner or later, in everyone's life, something horrible will happen and it'll hit them hard because they were too busy being happy to prepare themselves for it. Whereas I, on the other hand, have spent so long being miserable that nothing could possibly make me feel worse. But who could understand this? Not Adam, unfortunately. Not James. Not my family. I miss Sam. She's the only one I could talk to right now. But I can't. I can't possibly ask for her help. She's a kid, for God's sake. Adam isn't very good at comforting me. It seems that every time I feel bad, he's feeling worse and so I end up looking after him. It's not fair, really. It's nice to feel needed and I know I usually manage to make him feel better, but what about me? If I can't rely on my own boyfriend, who can I rely on? The other day, he asked me why I had a picture of the Two Fat Ladies in my purse. I couldn't believe he'd been looking through something as personal as my bloody purse! He said it was because he was looking for some change for the bus. I had to explain to him that when I looked at the picture it put me off eating and so it helped me control my weight. I was so embarrassed. And what did he do? He just laughed and said I was mad again. And he really doesn't understand how hard it is for me to be around him when he's eating chocolate, biscuits or anything remotely nice. He always offers me some and I have to say no despite my urge to take the whole thing off him and scoff it down. I've told him many times, but he says he's too polite not to share. So I tell him that the polite thing to do would be not to eat these in front of me in the first place and he argues that we spend too much time together for him to go without sugar.

Soon I won't even be able to talk to John. I've decided to leave the programme. If I don't, they'll kick me out anyway. I don't think it's helping me. I hate the group sessions. Renee was right – I can't talk about anything to do with Adam whilst he's in the same room. And since he's been in the group for longer than me, it makes sense for me to go. I'll be fine – I've lived over twenty-one years without therapy, I can manage another few decades. I doubt I'll try to kill myself again; there's probably a reason why I didn't succeed the first time. Or second rather, if you count my attempt with herbal pills. I haven't worked out what the actual reason is yet, but I'll find out eventually. Maybe it's Adam. If I hadn't done what I did, I'd never had met him. Not that I'm particularly grateful for that at the moment, but hopefully things will get better. Maybe the pills will help. They must be starting to have an effect soon, for Christ's sake. The only time I feel anything is when I'm drunk; but now, I'm not drunk the way I used to be. I feel light headed and dizzy. The other day, a friend of Adam's was having a house party, we were all sitting outside and this girl had been talking to me for at least an hour about god knows what, when I started feeling really sick. But I couldn't tell her to stop because every time I tried to interrupt her she'd pretend she didn't hear me. And after a while, I just couldn't keep it in anymore. So I jumped out of my chair and ran to the bathroom, treading on some flowers on the way. I could hear some people laughing and Guy, Adam's friend, screaming "Mind the flowers!" and I was so embarrassed. When I came back everyone asked me if I was OK, except for Adam. He didn't say anything until we'd left. He didn't want his beloved friends to think he was an arsehole.

"I can't believe you did that. I'm so embarrassed!"

"Don't you think I am? And I'm fine, by the way, thanks for asking!"

"You didn't seem fine. Why did you have to drink so much?"

"I drank the same amount you did!"

"Maybe you did, but I wasn't half as drunk as you were."

"Bullshit! Everyone was drunk!"

"But everyone didn't throw up in Guy's bathroom, did they?"

"So what? He'll get over it! You don't need to have a go at me, I've told you, I already feel crap about it."

"You shouldn't drink so much."

"It was an accident. And since when do you care how much I drink? You're the one who has beer for breakfast!"

"That only happened a couple of times. At least I know my limits."

"How many times have I had to look after you when you were pissed? How many times have you been in tears, telling me how much you hate yourself! Do you actually think you're fun when you're in that state?"

"At least I don't make a fool of myself! And I don't make you feel stupid in front of your friends!" I could have said so much about this, but there was no point. I've learnt that when he's in this frame of mind, the more I argue and try to defend myself, the more he'll get wound up and argue back. So I let him insult me and remind me what a horrible person I am. But when I start crying and tell him I want to go home by myself, it suddenly changes. I'm not such a bitch anymore. I'm the woman of his life, whom he's upset because he's an idiot and if I leave him he's going to kill himself because he feels so bad about hurting me. And when I say that I won't leave him, I'm just going to spend the night on my own because I need to have some time alone, he threatens to cut himself. And I can't go home knowing I'll be responsible for dozens of scars on his arms.

So I let him come home with me, we do things, he tells me he loves me, then falls asleep ... and I'm left once again to stare at the wall until dawn, wishing it hadn't happened. I still don't enjoy it. Sometimes I say no, but he persists, so I give in. At least he's always gentle. But I haven't had an orgasm for months. He tried at first, but I told him not to bother. I think it's got worse since I started the pills. We have sex because he wants to, and because I thrive to have at least a hint of normality in my life. What kind of relationship is one without sex? Friendship. And I wouldn't let my friends sleep in my bed or insult me when they're drunk. I do that myself well enough. I never thought I'd let him do it though. I really feel like I've let myself down. When we started going out, he was so different. He never stopped saying nice things, holding me and making me laugh. He was nice. Now I feel like whatever I do is wrong. He's so moody. I keep reminding myself that he's mentally ill and I cling on to the hope that one day things will be better. I told him I needed time alone, but he doesn't understand. Whenever I'm not with him, he texts me every five minutes. I can't breathe. That's why tonight, I told him I was with James; and turned my phone off.

****

Today's my last session with John. I struggle to fight the tears when I tell him I'm not coming back. He doesn't seem to acknowledge it. But there's no way around it: I've been promoted, I have to work everyday. I have no time for therapy. "We can't just let you go, he says. We have to discuss the alternatives." But there are no alternatives! "This promotion, how do you feel about it? It seems to have just come out of the blue … Last week you didn't appear too confident about your job." He knows I'm lying. He can see right through me. So I tell him. I burst into tears and tell him the whole story. He had his suspicions, apparently.

"Why didn't you say anything?"

"Because it wasn't my place to. It had to come from you."

"Well I can hardly stay now, can I?"

"We can't just throw you out. We don't want either of you to go."

"But what are you going to do? We can't go on as if nothing had happened!"

"Clearly not. I'll have to speak to the other therapists." He leaves it at that, and now I have to tell Adam that I might just have ruined his programme as well as mine. Something will change, but we won't know what until they tell us. Adam isn't going to like this.

"Aren't you going to say anything?"

"I don't know what to say. I just can't believe you told him."

"I had to. He didn't believe my story!"

"Well you obviously didn't tell it right."

"He's a therapist! He's going to know if I lie to him!"

"We've been lying for weeks!"

"He knew. He just didn't want to tell us."

"Bullshit. And even if he did, he could have kept on not telling us."

"Aren't you happy that I won't get chucked out?"

"We don't know that yet. We don't know anything. They could throw us both out and then what?"

"They won't. I'm sure they can put me in a different group or something."

"It's more complicated than that."

"How do you know? Are you a therapist?"

"Don't take that tone with me!"

"Oh for god's sake, stop being so childish."

"Childish? You've just ruined my only chance of getting better!"

"No, you're ruining it yourself by being such an arsehole!" That shuts him up, as though I'd said something he'd never thought of. He finishes his coffee, gets up and walks out of the cafe where we were supposed to have lunch, just as the waitress comes with our plates. I smile awkwardly, eat a few leaves of my salad and pay. Thankfully it's 2:00pm in the middle of the week, so the place is nearly empty. I hate arguing in the middle of a crowd. I had to tell him in public, because if we'd been alone his reaction could have been far worse. I'm annoyed, but hopeful. Maybe I'll stay in therapy after all. I walk out of the cafe and jump. Standing in front of me, in a large white flannel dress, is Naomi.

"Oh my god! Hi Mel!"

"Hi. How... are you?"

"I'm... good. You?"

"G...good. What a... coincidence!"

"Yes! It certainly is." And then, the obvious awkward silence. "Well... See you then."

"See you." I walk away, but soon after I hear my name. "Do you fancy a drink?"

It's strange to see her after so long. I never thought I would speak to her again. And yet, there we are, having coffee, talking about all and nothing, like the old times.

"So... Tell me. What have you been doing?"

"Well, I passed my exams and now I work for a firm of Chartered Accountants. It's going well so far. But I'm going to be out of work for a while soon", she says, stroking her stomach.

"Why? Are you ill?"

"Not exactly. I'm prenant." Bloody hell. I did think the dress was a bit too big.

"Oh. Wow. Err... That's..."

"A shock? Yeah. Tell me about it. But anyway, what have you been doing?" She asks, clearly trying to change the subject. I would have thought she'd be over the moon.

"You know. This and that."

"Come on, Mel! I haven't seen you for months! You must have things to tell me."

"I... I haven't been very well." I say after a long pause.

"No? What's happened?"

"I became quite depressed. Remember that guy I met on the internet?"

"Simon?"

"Yes. Well, I met him. And it really upset me."

"Why?"

"It made me realise how bad things were. I was hopeless. So I did something very, very silly."

"You didn't kill him, did you?" I can't help letting a giggle out.

"No. But I tried to kill... me." She stares at me silently, her mouth wide open, as though she was going to swallow the earth.

"Oh my god. Mel, that's awful. When did that happen?"

"Shortly after we stopped talking. But I'm better now, see? I'm still standing."

"How... how did you do it?"

"I took some pills", I say as casually as I can, "And... this." I show her my wrists.

"Oh."

"I don't know why, really, but I did it in a park. So someone found me before it was too late. They rang an ambulance, I was taken to hospital where I got told off for throwing up, then I was sent to a mental ward", I say in one breath. I'd been dying to tell someone sane for a long time.

"A mental ward?" she repeats. "How long were you there for?"

"Five days. It felt more like five years."

"What was it like?"

"Awful. I couldn't shower properly, I wasn't allowed to go out... They wouldn't even let me charge my phone."

"It must have been so scary. I can't imagine it, really. That's the kind of thing you'd only expect to see in films."

"It was real."

"So... What now?"

"I'm in therapy. But I might not stay for very long because I've started seeing a guy in my group."

"Really? You have a boyfriend?" She clears her throat, probably realising she sounded too obviously surprised. "That's great!"

"Yeah. It's... great."

"What's he like?" The only thing that comes to mind is a four-letter word starting with c.

"He's... nice."

"And? Come on, what does he look like? What does he do?"

"I used to think he looked like Ewan McGregor in Train Spotting. But now, he's more like the character in Star Wars. And he doesn't do anything."

"Nothing at all?"

"He writes."

"Ooh, a writer! What's he done?"

"Nothing you'd heard of. He hasn't been published yet. And I haven't seen him do anything since we got together."

"Oh. So, how does he get paid?"

"He doesn't. He's on benefits. And his parents give him pocket money."

"Oh", she repeats. "I see. Well, maybe not for long though, I mean, he might get published soon, right?" I can tell she's trying hard to be nice about it; but she's never had a good opinion of people like him.

"So, is it a boy or a girl?" I ask in a desperate attempt to change subject.

"I don't know. I don't want to."

"How does George feel about it? I assume it's his?" She laughs, then lets out a sigh.

"It certainly is. He wasn't too happy at first. Neither was I, to be honest. But we've both got used to the idea now. It does compromise things a bit… a lot, actually. But it's too late now."

"Well, there are different options, you know. If you don't want to keep it…"

"No! It's… OK. It's going to be fine. I've always wanted kids anyway, you know that. I just didn't think I'd have one so soon. With my first-ever boyfriend. We're moving in together next month. We have to." I couldn't imagine living with Adam. I'd end up killing him. If he didn't kill me first. "Anyway, I should get going. My lunch break's almost over." I've never known how to end a discussion, but this time it's even worse. What should I say? Nice to see you? Good luck with everything? Can I call you? But thankfully, she speaks first.

"I've still got your number. Maybe I could ring you sometime?"

"Yes. That'd be nice."

****

My dilemma of the day is that next week, it's my mother's 50th. Not only does that mean that I have to see her and the whole family, including some cousins I barely know and an uncle I hate, but she's invited Adam. I had to tell her about him eventually. Apparently, they're 'all looking forward to meeting him', and if I don't bring him they'll think I made him up. I'm sure she only invited him to check I hadn't. Thing is, I slightly lied to her about Adam and he doesn't know. I told her his first book was about to be published and that he had a cat – hence the cuts, so if anyone notices them they won't freak out. I don't think he'd mind so much about that, but he wouldn't understand about the book. He thinks it's OK to have been on benefits for over a year, even though he's perfectly capable of working. The only reason he doesn't is that he's lazy. He says the one job he'd consider doing would be working in a video shop, but he won't go to Blockbuster because "they wear stupid uniforms" and the other shops are too far away. Frankly, sometimes when I look at him I feel better about myself. My other concern is that Christmas is only a few weeks away and I've no idea what to get him. I want to ask him, but I'm scared he'll tell me off for a) not knowing him enough to guess and b) being too lazy to think of ideas. But I also don't want to risk buying him something he won't like, because then he'll have a go at me for wasting money. I might just wait a while to see if he mentions anything and if not I'll have to rack my brain and suffer the consequences. My mother's not the only one who's been bugging me about meeting Adam; James has been going on and on about how offended he is that I haven't introduced him yet. I'm worried he thinks I'm embarrassed of him because he's gay. But I can hardly admit to anyone that I'm embarrassed of my own boyfriend, can I? So I've given up trying to make up excuses and they're finally meeting tonight. I had to practically beg Adam to come out, as he said he wasn't feeling "sociable". When does he ever, that's what I'd like to know. I struggled to find a venue; Adam hates Whetherspoons, and James won't go anywhere that doesn't play chart music. In the end, on James's advice, we go to a place called The Observatory, off Tottenham Court Road. The music isn't "too bad", in Adam's words, but James omitted to tell me that it was a gay bar.

"It's not, really! Look at these two, they're a straight couple, aren't they?"

"James... That's a woman."

"No way! Really?"

"I saw her coming out of the ladies' toilets."

"Oh. Sorry. Well, it's not supposed to be gay. I've seen straight people here before. What's wrong with that, anyway?"

"Nothing. It's just... Adam's not used to these places."
"So? There's a first time for everything. And no one's going to jump on him!"

"I know. Don't worry about it. Let's just get some drinks. What do you want?" I ask Adam when he comes back from the loo.

"Lager, please." He sits at an empty table and gets up again shortly after to browse the magazines on a shelf.

"So, what do you think?" I ask James, fearing the answer.

"Give us a chance, darling! We haven't spoken yet. But I can see the attraction, he definitely looks like Ewan McGregor; a grungy Ewan McGregor." Grungy? I never thought I'd one day go out with a "grunge". I never dreamt in a million years of being associated with that word.

"What are you reading?" I ask Adam as we sit down.

"Nothing. They're all gay magazines." He replies dryly.

"We didn't know it was a gay bar. Sorry", I say forcing a smile. He shrugs.

"So, Adam, Mel tells me you're a writer?"

"Yeah. But I haven't been published yet."

"What d'you write about?"

"Various things." We both wait for him to elaborate, but he doesn't add any more.

"He's written a book based on his experiences, more or less. And also a couple of plays!" I intervene, trying to sound enthusiastic – or proud, maybe.

"Oh, excellent."

"And you work for Virgin?"

"That's right. So, if you ever need CDs or DVDs, let me know and I'll get you a staff discount!"

"Thanks, but I don't shop at Virgin. I only go to independent shops."

"Really? Why is that?" And so Adam goes on about how mainstream mega stores are slowly swallowing all the small businesses and how, eventually, there'll only be one music store, one restaurant chain and one brand for everything and we'll all have turned into robots. I used to be fascinated by his ideologies; but right now, I just want to slap him.

"If you'll excuse me, I've got to powder my nose", James says as he gets up and heads for the toilets.

"Are you OK?" I ask as calmly as I can.

"Yeah, why?"

"Because I feel like you're trying to ruin the evening."

"You what?" He smirks.

"Why are you being so rude? He's only trying to make conversation!"

"I'm not being rude. I'm making conversation back. You're the one who left me by myself looking like a prat while you two were at the bar!"

"I was buying your drink! You're so ungrateful. Can you at least try to be nicer to him?" But James comes back before he can answer. He sits silently for a while, whilst James and I discuss his latest fling; then, suddenly, he gets up.

"I think I'm going to head home; I'm quite tired. Nice to meet you." He waves at James and leaves, without giving me the glimpse of an eye.

"Well, he's certainly one of a kind!" James says after an uncomfortable silence.

"Is that your tactful way of saying you hate him?"

"Of course I don't hate him. I just find him a bit… scary. Does he treat you well?"

"Yes! Most of the time it's… great. He has a few issues, that's all."

"Do you love him?"

"Yes… I think so."

"And does he?"

"Yes. As far as I know, anyway."

"Tell me something. I get the feeling that I'm not the only one who's scared of him."

"Me? No! Don't be silly. I'm not a battered woman, James."

"You don't need to be beaten up to have wounds, darling", he says quietly, pointing at his head.

"Cut the cheese", I say jokingly. "I'm fine, honest. Anyway, what are you going to do about Dave?"

Ten missed calls and no messages. He always does that. As I go home, I expect to see him sat outside my door; but surprisingly, he's not there. As soon as I walk into my room, however, the phone rings.

"Can I come over?" He sounds quite upset, so I let him. "You didn't even check that I was OK when I left."

"You said you were tired! What did you want me to do, run after you?"

"Well, yes, actually!"

"I don't believe it. Do you realise how juvenile this is?"

"So what?"

"So this was a chance for you to meet one of my only friends and you've made a fool of yourself!"

"As if I give a shit what he thinks!"

"I do! He's my friend, he's part of my life!" This is exactly what I was like with Naomi when I met George. How did she put up with me for so long?

"Maybe if we'd been in a normal place I wouldn't have felt so uncomfortable! All the men were staring at me."

"Don't flatter yourself. They were probably wondering why you looked so bloody miserable!"

"Do you know what I was doing while you and your little token gay friend were fooling around?" Not that again. I'm so bored of hearing it.

"Don't try to make me feel guilty for wanting to have a good time. I need that time! And what do you mean, token gay friend?" He shakes his head, picks up his jacket and opens the door. "Don't do this. You can't just walk out on me whenever things don't go your way!" I throw myself on the bed, tears pouring down.

"I'm sorry", he says, closing the door.

"I'm so sick of this. Why can't we have a normal, happy relationship, like everyone else?" He sits next to me, and runs his fingers through my hair.

"Because we're not normal. We're not like everyone else. That's why we're made for each other. No one else understands what's in our heads." I don't know whether he's trying to comfort me, or convince me, or himself, that we're not wasting our time together and making things worse for each other. Either way, it's not working.

"I just want to sleep right now."

"OK. Can I stay?"

"Yes." I bury myself in his arms, as though, for a few hours, they could protect me from everything, including him. I lay there, drained but unable to rest.

"My mother wants to meet you. Do you think you can pretend to be normal for one evening?"

****

He looks good. He's had his hair cut, he's shaved and put on some clean and sensible clothes. He looks a different man. The man I fell for. I didn't want to go out tonight; I wanted to keep him all to myself. But we're meeting my mother and a dozen other people in "Simply Nico", my mother's favourite restaurant, and hopefully he'll be on his best behaviour.

"Mum, dad, this is Adam."

"Hello Adam, it's so nice to meet you at last!" My mother says, a big smile on her face.

"Same to you, Mrs Stevenson."
"Please, call me Eunice."

"Well done Mel, he's gorgeous!" Jenny whispers as we sit down. My cousins Linda and Robert arrive shortly after, with my aunt Di and uncle Patrick, whom I've hated since the day I caught him talk dirty on the phone to someone who wasn't Di; I told my mother but she never believed me. There are also a couple of my Mum's friends and a rather handsome young man, who apparently works with my mother sometimes. When she introduces us, he shakes my hand. Everyone orders starters except me, so I sit staring at my empty plate while they all eat. I'm starving, but I'd feel stupid ordering a salad for starters and another one for the main course. From time to time, I catch the young man looking at me and when our eyes meet, he smiles.

"What do you think of him?" Jenny asks when he goes to the gents.

"He's alright. But he seems a bit young for me! And I have Adam, remember?"

"I wasn't talking about you, silly!" She blushes.

"Oh, I see. Well, yes, he seems very pleasant. And cute, too."

"Do you think I stand a chance?"

"Yeah. I don't see why not." I feel slightly jealous, somehow, as if I wanted to keep his eyes for myself only. Adam seems very outgoing for once; he talks to my parents a lot. I think they like him. And they don't seem to mind that he's not working; apparently my mother thinks it's amazing that he's written books and plays. But as we finish the main course, I nearly die.

"Have you seen much of Naomi, lately?" My mother asks.

"I saw her last week. She's pregnant."

"Is she really? Does she know the sex?"

"No. She doesn't want to yet."

"You didn't tell me about that", Adam intervenes.

"Really? I must have forgotten."

"How often do you see her?" He continues. What's it to him anyway?

"Only that once. I'll tell you about it later", I whisper. I never told mother we'd stopped seeing each other.

"So, how does she feel about it?" My mother asks.

"She's OK, I think. She's moving in with her boyfriend soon."

"Well, that's very wise. I'll tell you who else is pregnant: Elise! Can you believe it?" Elise is my Mum's neighbour's daughter and she's only a year older than Jenny.

"Maybe it's contagious", my uncle butts in. I hadn't realised he'd been listening. He gives me a meaningful look, which I find particularly out of place.

"No, not me." I say sharply.

"But one day, obviously", Adam says, and I jump.

"Oh really?" My mother says with apparent delight. I don't like this. "How many children would you want, Adam?"

"Two, maybe three. Girls, hopefully."

"Well that's wonderful, isn't it, Melanie?" I don't believe this! What the hell is going on? He's never discussed having children with me!

"So, when can we expect the first one?" Patrick asks with a big smirk on his face.

"Well, not just now, but maybe in a couple of years; you know, once we…"

"Excuse me!" I stop him straight, "But don't I get a say in this?"

"Sorry dear, I thought you two had talked about it already", my mother says, looking somewhere between confused and amused.

"There's obviously been a misunderstanding. I'm… not remotely ready." Everyone is staring at me now. I've never been so embarrassed in my whole life. I can't believe he's thinking of having children. How does he expect us to look after kids when we can't even look after ourselves?

"Your family's lovely", he says as we leave the restaurant.

"How could you do this to me?" I'm trying hard not to break down in the middle of the street.

"What are you talking about?"

"You know full well! You had no right to start discussing my future with my parents!"

"I wasn't discussing your future, I was discussing ours!"

"Adam, when you talk about something that's going to be inside my body for nine months, that's my future!"

"Can you calm down? People are staring."

"Since when do you care? You make a scene practically every time we're out!"

"That's not true."

"Whatever. I don't want you to stay with me tonight. I want to be alone."

"I haven't got my keys, remember? I left them in your room."

"Well, you can pick them up and go."

"What?" He laughs, "You know how hard it is to get from your house to mine, especially at night!"

"Fine, I'll order you a cab then."

"Don't you think you're over reacting?"

"Over reacting?" I'm fuming. "You made a fool of me in front of my whole family!"

"Aren't you pleased that I have plans for us?"

"I can't believe you're even considering having children right now. We're mad, remember? Don't you think that it could somehow affect our abilities to be parents?"

"But we're in therapy. The whole point of it is to get better!"

"Look, Adam. I don't want children. I never have and never will." He looks thrown.

"That's what you think right now, but maybe in a couple of years time you'll change your mind."

"I doubt it. But if I do, it'll be my own decision. And I won't have you, or anyone else, put words into my mouth." I get into my room, hand him his keys and dial a cab office. But he takes the receiver off me and puts it down.

"Can we talk about this first?"

"There's nothing to talk about. I told you, I need time alone."

"But we can't leave things like this!"

"Look, I'm exhausted. Right now, I just want to forget about tonight."

"I'm sorry for upsetting you. I shouldn't have discussed such personal things with your family."

"Thanks. But I still want to be alone. Apologising doesn't take things away."

"What else do you want me to do? I can't turn back time!" It's like talking to a brick wall.

"All I want you to do right now is leave me alone. You're not making it any better by arguing with me."

"I'm not arguing with you, I'm trying to sort things out!"

"If you want to sort things out, then please, leave!" I say sharply. I pick up the receiver again, but he grabs my hand, quite firmly.

"Don't."

"Let go! You're hurting me." But he squeezes harder.

"Then don't do this."

"What do you think you're doing? Let go of me. You're pathetic!" A second after, I'm on the floor. He slapped me. Really, really hard.

"Oh God. I'm so sorry."

"Get out. Get out or I'll scream!" As he leaves, I burst into tears. I hadn't been hit since I was a child. "I'll never hurt you", he said not long ago. I get up, wash my face and put some music on. Not long after, there's a knock on the door.

"Are you still there?" I shout from inside, shaking. "I told you to go away!"

"Mel? It's me, James." I open the door, trying hard to smile.

"Hiya. What's up?" I say casually.

"Are you OK?" He quickly glances around my room."

"Yes, I'm fine. Why?"

"You didn't sound fine a minute ago. I heard some shouting, so I thought I'd come down to see if you needed help."

"Help? No, thanks. I'm good."

"You're all flushed. And your cheek's red. What's happened?" I sigh.

"We had an argument. But it's OK now."

"You keep saying. Did he hurt you?"

"No! Well... Yes, I suppose. Just once."

"Just once? That doesn't make it OK! How often does he do that?"

"It was the first time. And the last."

"Yes, because you're going to dump him."

"I... don't know about that."

"Are you serious? Mel, the guy's assaulted you!"

"I wouldn't go that far. It was just a slap."

"So what? Next thing you're going to tell me you deserved it!"

"Maybe I did. I don't really know anymore..."

"Darling, whatever you did, he shouldn't have hit you. If anyone did that to me, I'd go straight to the police!" I smile.

"I don't think a little slap is an arrestable offence."

"It's not the first time you guys have argued though, is it?"

"How do you know?"

"My room's above yours, remember?" How embarrassing. That means he's probably heard us have sex as well!

"I didn't want to say anything because I didn't feel it was my place. But he's gone too far this time."

"But... it's not really his fault. He's got issues. He's in therapy." I take a deep breath. "And so am I. That's where we met."

"You're in therapy? Why?"

"Because I'm not well. It's a long story. I get depressed sometimes. and he does too." A big part of me expects him to run off and never speak to me again; but he doesn't.

"Darling, why did you never tell me?"
"I was too embarrassed."

"Don't be! We've all got issues. But that doesn't give him the right to walk over you. You can do so much better for yourself."

"I doubt anyone normal would ever want to be with me."

"Honey, depression doesn't make you abnormal! It's very common, you know."

"Really? I don't know anyone who has it, apart from us and the people in the programme."

"I know a few. The bottom line is, he's not good to you."

"But I'm scared to be alone. I got used to his company. And he's really nice, most of the time."

"But what about the few times when he's not? What if one day he hits you too hard and you end up like Nicky Cartwright?" I hadn't thought of that. I shiver.

"Even if I did break up with him, it wouldn't make things any better. He'd probably kill himself. He told me." He rolls his eyes.

"That's the oldest trick in the book. It's called emotional blackmail."

"He sounded pretty serious. I couldn't live with myself if he did it!"

"I'm sure we'll find a nice and gentle way to break up with him. And I know a few gorgeous young men who'd probably love to spend some time with you!"

"I thought you weren't talking to me anymore", he says as he lets me into his lounge. He looks even scruffier than usual and from the smell I'm guessing he hasn't had a wash nor changed his clothes in a while.

"It's only been a few days. I needed time to think." The reason why I'm doing this in his house is because it would have been unfair to make him come to mine, and he would have probably made a fool of himself and embarrassed me in a public place. James is picking me up in an hour, just in case it goes horribly wrong and he has to rescue me.

"Drink?" He offers me a beer, after taking a sip of his. It's not even 11:00am and he only got up a few minutes ago.

"No, thanks." He sits on his sofa and I sit on the chair in front of him. I try hard not to show how terrified I am. I don't want to hurt him.

"I don't really know how to do this... or what to say, really." I had prepared a whole speech, but now it all seems very tacky.

"You want to dump me."

"I wouldn't say I want to; but I think it's for the best. You must realise how hard it's been recently. It just hasn't been working."

"Fine. Go away. You never gave a shit about me anyway."

"That's really unfair! I've tried so hard to support you. I've always been there when you needed me, and who was there for me?"

"You're so ungrateful. Didn't I come to your house at three in the morning because you couldn't sleep?"

"That happened once, Adam. It hardly compares to what you made me put up with. I haven't come here for an argument, anyway. I just thought I'd be considerate and do this face to face rather than sending you a text message. I'll see myself out." I expect him to run after me, but he doesn't. Did I really mean that little to him that he won't even try to patch things up or apologise? Or maybe he's about to kill himself! I should go back in and check. But I can't! I can't go back there. James is right, it's emotional blackmail. I get my phone out of my bag and dial Renee's number. As she picks up, I can't contain the tears.

"Renee? I've split up with Adam and I'm really worried he might try to do something stupid. Please, could you check that he's OK?"

"I'm sure he'll be fine, darling. You did the right thing." James hands me a tissue and gives me a hug. "You'll feel much better soon. Trust me. Plenty of fish in the sea and we'll go fishing them together! The first thing we have to do is review your wardrobe. No offence, but you've got a Prunella Scales - Tesco advert look going on here!"

"There's nothing wrong with my clothes, thank you very much."

"Not if you're sixty, no! But boys want to see tits and arses!"

"I don't want anyone to see my tits and arse! I don't even like seeing them myself."

"Well, we'll work on that. By the time I'm finished with you, you'll be gagging to be a Page 3 girl!"

"I don't see it happen. To be honest, I don't see much happen. I feel like my head is empty." I take a couple of long sips of my drink and pinch my leg.

"Are you still popping pills?" I jump.

"What?"

"The Prozac thingy."

"Oh. Yes. But I'm starting to think I'm wasting my time. And money."

"I don't know much about anti-depressants, but surely there's only so much they can do. If your mum dies, she dies and I don't think there's anything that can make you not sad about it."

"But my mother's not dead", I say, confused.

"You know what I mean. You can't expect them to turn you into a different person. You have to do that yourself. And I'm going to help you."

Chapter 7

James opens my wardrobe and lets out a cry.

"Bloody hell! It's worse than I thought. OK, first of all, who died? There's not a hint of colour here!"

"Black makes me look thin."

"OK, these", he says picking up a couple of jumpers, "say to me 'Fuck off and don't even consider talking to me.'"

"Really? To me they just say 'Hi, I'm a black jumper'."

"Very funny, smart arse. Your clothes are a reflection of your mind."

"Where did you get that from? Spiritualism for Dummies?"

"I'm a gay man, I know these things. Just trust me."

"I don't want to look like a tart. I like my jumpers!"

"You won't look like a tart. You will look like a gorgeous, confident young woman."

"But I'm not."

"We'll work on that." He takes the elastic band out of my hair and combs it with his hands.

"Much better already. Now, let's go do some shopping."

He takes me to Oxford Street and I daren't tell him I hate every inch of that place; I figure the less I say, the quicker we'll be done and I can go back to being a boring spinster. He makes me try on the most ridiculously tarty outfits that even Jordan wouldn't be seen dead in... and threatens to pay for them himself if I don't. So I end up with three miniskirts, four silky-type vests, three pairs of "trendy" tights, as he puts it and a pair of knee-high boots. Then we move on to makeup. Mascara, lipstick, eyeliner, nothing I didn't have already, but apparently they were "completely the wrong colour". But the worse was yet to come.

"We're nearly done. We've just got to check out some underwear."

"What? No way. I'm not buying knickers with you!"

"Why not? It's not like I'm going to perve!"

"You're still a man. A person! I wouldn't even buy them with Naomi!"

"You're insane."

"Yes, and?"

"And we're still going in." He grabs my arm and drags me towards La Senza.

"No," I say half giggling, "I'm not going in!"

"Fine. Wait here." He looks at my waist and says to himself, but loud enough so I hear, "Size 10". I wait outside, nervous and amused and he comes back out after less than five minutes with a big bag. "Want to see what's inside?"

"I'm not sure!" I open the bag and dig out two velvet thongs, two bras and a lacy corset.

"Oh my god."

"Nice isn't it?"

"You're crazier than I am. These must have cost a fortune! I don't have the money!"

"I'm not asking you for any money. Let's say they're early Christmas presents."

"I can't accept them. This is probably a week's worth of your wage!"

"Don't worry about it. Trust me, it's nothing. Now, I'm exhausted. Let's go have a coffee." He points at the Starbucks across the street.

"Adam would kill me if he knew I was here", I say as I take a sip of coffee.

"I could think of better reasons for him wanting to kill you." I frown. "Sorry, that wasn't funny. Have you heard from him?"

"No. I don't know if that's a good or a bad thing."

"Definitely a good one. If anything had happened you would have been told."

"I guess so. But just because he's not dead doesn't mean he's OK."

"Just concentrate on yourself. He has his friends to look after him."

"That's the thing, I don't think he does. He used to tell me I was the only one who understood him."

"And he probably said that to all his previous girlfriends. No offence, of course", he says tapping on my arm. "He's a big boy, he'll get over it. So, are you excited about your new look?"

"Frightened, rather. I don't think I have the guts to wear all this."

"Oh yes you do, young lady. Are you working on Sunday?"

"Don't think so, why?"

"Good. We're going clubbing on Saturday, in your new clothes."

"I… don't know about that."

"Why not? What have you got planned that could possibly be more exciting?"

"Nothing, but I could think of a million things more exciting than clubbing. You know how much I hate clubs. They're like meat markets."

"Well, yes, I suppose they are, but you'll be safe where I'm taking you. We're going to a gay club."

"And how would I get in? I told you, I'm not planning to become a lesbian."

"You don't need to. You'll get in, you're my fag hag!"

****

"My god, this is huge!" I cry as I walk into James's room. I expected it to be the same size as mine, but it's at least twice as big. I wonder how he can afford it.

"I need space, I have a lot of junk!"

"Well it's… very nice. The rent must be extortionate."

"It's alright. What would you like to drink? Red or white? Or beer?"

"White, please. I need help… I don't know what to wear." I throw the pile of clothes I was holding on his bed and sigh.

"Let's sort you out." He scans them one by one, pulling faces. "This, and this." He picks up the short denim skirt and black vest. "And the diamond tights."

"Very eighties", I say grimacing.

"No, very you. Put these on, I'm going to shake my lettuce."

"You what?" He laughs.

"I'm going for a pee." When he comes back, he does my hair and make up. "Amazing. You should be on the catwalk." I look at myself in the mirror and for the first time since my mother got me into a Pocahontas costume when I was nine, I quite like what I see.

"Is this really me?"

"It certainly is. How do you feel?" I smile.

"Rather good."

"Come one, finish your drink and let's go shake our arses!"

The queue is huge, the people are loud and my tights are itchy. On top of that, I drank half a bottle of wine on the way and I'm desperate for a pee. James makes every possible effort to humour me, but I'm not in the mood. I want to go home and hide in my bed.

"What's wrong?"

"Nothing", I reply, not wanting his friends to think I'm a miserable bag.

"Come on."

"It's just weird being here, in these clothes. I feel like a teenager. Except that I never dressed like this."

"You'll get used to it. You're going to have a great night, I promise." You shouldn't promise things you have no power over, I want to say. After about an hour of queuing, we finally get in and I rush to the toilets; but the place is so big that it takes me another five minutes to find them. When I come out, I make my way to the bar, where James was supposed to wait for me; but he's nowhere to be seen. I get myself a drink and look around. The place is packed with muscled, happy looking men; it's as though I were caught in a Top Shop catalogue. I wonder what they all have to be so cheerful about. I don't think I've ever seen a gay man frown.

"Having fun?" A woman next to me asks. She's wearing baggy trousers, a cotton vest, has short hair and a big ring in her nose.

"Sorry, I'm not gay", I reply, anxious.

"I was only trying to be friendly", she snaps, obviously offended, and walks off. I don't belong here. Not just because I'm straight, but because they all seem to share this bright and happy gene that I clearly don't have. I finish my drink quickly and head for the cloakroom.

"Not leaving already, are you?" Someone asks as I start queuing. This is quite embarrassing; everyone else is obviously dropping their coats off and I'm picking mine up.

"Well... yes, I am."

"Why? It's only just started?" For god's sake. What's it to him anyway?

"I'm not feeling well."

"You probably just need a drink!" Looks like he's already had his share.

"Come on! We'll look after you!" His friend says, and they grab my arms. I must really look like the perfect fag hag. I let them take me to the bar, where they buy me a drink I quickly down, so I get them one as well. After finishing the second one, I feel a bit better.

"Let's have a dance!" I follow them onto the dance floor, not wanting to be left alone again. The songs are surprisingly good and I enjoy a few dances with my new "friends", who bring me more and more alcohol every time my glass is empty. After a while and a lot of alcohol, I manage to relax and rather enjoy myself.

"Mel! Where the hell have you been?" James says, appearing out of nowhere.

"Hi! I thought you'd abandoned me! This is Mark and Andrew. Come dance with us!" A few moments later, I'm in the centre of a circle of men who, one by one, have a short dance with me. For the first time in my life, I feel popular.

"We should get our coats soon", James says suddenly.

"What? Already?"

"It's nearly five! The club's going to close in a minute."

"Nearly five?"

"Yes", James says laughing. "Someone's clearly had a good time! Come on, we can come back next weekend if you really want to. Andrew's coming back with us by the way", he says a big smile on his face. I get my coat reluctantly and we head for the bus stop. I don't really remember the journey home nor getting into bed and wake up the next morning grateful that I fell asleep without hearing my friends shag.

****

I'm starting to like my new look. People at work were really shocked at first. "I didn't know you had legs!" someone even said. A lot of people have complimented me and now I definitely feel more confident. Well, not so confident that I could start a random conversation with some stranger, but still, it's progress. I go out with James quite a lot and everyone I meet seems to like me! I never thought I'd see the day. But John is really annoying me at the moment, he doesn't seem to appreciate that I'm finally happy.

"I'm a bit concerned about your alcohol intake. From what you've said, you seem to associate going out and socialising with getting drunk." So I tell him that I'm boring and quiet when I'm sober and the drinks make me more outgoing; but he thinks I should make an effort to be sociable without alcohol. Well, that's not going to happen. I tried once, but no one would talk to me and every time I tried to say something I got cut off. And everyone else drinks, so I can't be the only sober one. I've asked him for a diagnosis; at first he was quite reluctant, because apparently therapists don't like to do that. So I said that if there was something wrong with my body I'd expect to be told what it was and it was only fair that my mental health was treated the same way. He said he'd talk to his superior about it. I started in the new group yesterday; I felt quite uncomfortable, because I didn't know what they'd been told about me. And I don't think I could ever talk about Adam in case any of them knows him. Plus, the therapist is quite scary. He's called Wilfred, has big round glasses and blatantly wears a toupee. He looks more like a scientist than a counsellor. But I don't really care. Everything else in my life is good at the moment and I won't let them spoil it. The only thing I'm really stressed about is Christmas. It's now only a couple of weeks away and I haven't started my shopping. I'd told myself that I'd do it early this year, but I just didn't get around to it, what with everything that's been happening recently. Not only do I never know what to buy (my mother's answer to "What would everyone like for Christmas" is generally "Just your presence, dear"), but the worst is, I hate the shops during that period even more than usual. You hear the same tacky music everywhere, people are rushing around, shouting at their screaming kids who throw tantrums because they want everything they see, not to mention all the Santas and elves at every corner. It's draining. Since James hates it as much as me, we've decided to do our shopping together. We start our day with a couple of drinks, just to relax a bit before facing the storm. But we end up drinking much more than planned and I wander from one shop to another, not really sure what's going on around me or what I'm doing, so I don't actually buy anything at all. It occurs to me afterwards that James seems to have bought rather expensive presents; not that I have anything against generous people, but I can't imagine stacking up shelves in a music store paying enough to buy half of what he's got today, not to mention the underwear at La Senza. So unless he's won the lottery or his mum gives him pocket money, there's something dodgy going on.

"I knew you'd ask me sooner or later."

"Tell me then. Are you a drug dealer?"

"Drug dealer?" He laughs hard. "Do you really see me as a drug dealer?"

"Well, not really. But what then?"

"Don't judge me, OK?"

"I can't promise that."

"Then I can't tell you."

"Oh come on! You can't not tell me now. You know I'll get it out of you sooner or later."

"OK, OK." He takes deep breath.

"I'm an escort." For a moment, I stay speechless.

"You mean... you sleep with people for money?"

"Well, kind of, yeah."

"What do you mean, kind of? You either do or you don't!"

"Sometimes I do, sometimes I don't. Depends if I want to. Tell me you're not cross?"

"Cross? I'm more shocked than anything else. How can you do that to yourself? You sell your body!"

"I know. But it's really good money. I can't afford to live on five pounds an hour." I can't believe what I'm hearing.

"Then get a better job! It's not that hard you know, millions of people do it!"

"I haven't got any qualifications, I never went to uni."

"Neither did I. But I worked my way up."

"Well you're obviously more clever than I am."

"That's not what I meant. It's laziness."

"I'm not lazy. Just... insecure."

"So am I! But you shouldn't be. You're bright and young, you've got plenty of time to learn new skills."

"You know the only thing I really want to do is sing."

"Then imagine the day when you're famous and someone goes to the paper telling them you used to be a prostitute!"

"It's a risk I'm ready to take. Think about it: you get paid to have sex!"

"I know. That's my point! Don't you have any self respect?" He sighs.

"Don't go all righteous on me."

"How do you find your clients?"

"I've got an advert on the internet."

"And how often do you do it?"

"Depends. Once, twice a week, sometimes more, sometimes less. Oh, cheer up will you, it's not that bad. I haven't killed anyone."

"No, but one of them could kill you. Have you thought of the shit you could catch?"

"Of course I have! I'm not stupid. Look, I know it's not your thing. But as long as I'm happy, surely that's all that matters? Just be grateful for the lovely undies."

"Which you didn't have to give me."

"I know that. But I like spoiling my friends. And you needed them. Anyway, I haven't seen you use your new irresistible charms yet."

"That's because I don't have any. And who would I use them on? I can't exactly try to pick up gay men, can I."

"Let's go to a straight club then!"

"You'd go to a straight club?"

"Yes, why not? I can be straight." I let out a giggle.

"Sure. So you won't be wearing tight trousers and baby lotion then?"

"Absolutely not. I'll be butcher than Schwarzenegger."

I don't know why I said yes. I don't want to go to a straight club. I feel safe amongst gay men. There's no tension, no drama. They like me. Straight men don't. They'll think I look stupid and that I can't dance. But James promised me that if it's horrible, we can go to G.A.Y. Naomi recommended this place in Camden that plays disco; apparently it's the only club she and

George used to go to before she got pregnant. I haven't eaten anything today apart from an apple, so I could look a bit slimmer. We drank nearly two bottles of wine on the way, so I have to practically beg the bouncer to let us in. It's almost as big as the Astoria; as we walk towards the cloakroom, three men in white shirts smile at me.

"See? We've only been here two minutes and you've already pulled!"

"They were probably taking the piss."

"Oh, shut up you silly cow!" We drop off our coats and James drags me to the bar. Then he goes to the gents, so I sit on a stool at the counter. I down my drink and get another one, similar, so he doesn't notice. Not long after, one of the men in white shirts appears next to me. He has short dark hair and blue eyes, and quite a cute smile.

"Alright?"

"Yeah."

"Is that your boyfriend with you?" I laugh.

"James? No. More like my girlfriend", I say, rather proud of my joke. But I don't think he gets it.

"Pardon?"

"Nothing."

"D'you come here often?"

"No, it's my first time actually."

"Really? Oh well, if you need a guide, I'm all yours!" A guide in a nightclub? I hope he's not serious.

"Thanks, but I can look after myself."

"Sure, sorry. See, I'm not very good at chatting up girls. Especially when they're so gorgeous." I know it's really sleazy, but I'm enjoying it.

"I think you're doing quite well."

"Really? Do you want to dance, then?" Part of me kind of wants to; after all, he seems to like me, for some obscure reason! But a) I should wait for James and b) if I get up I might fall over and die of embarrassment. James comes back before I can form an answer.

"Who's your friend, then?" He asks, a big smile on his face. And then I realise that I don't actually know.

"I'll leave you to it", the cute guy says before I get a chance to ask him.

"You can stay!" I say, rather angry at James for interrupting us.

"I should go back to my mates. Nice meeting you." He waves and leaves, giving James a disapproving look.

"What's his problem?" James asks, obviously offended.

"I'm not sure. Maybe you scared him off, you big butch."

"Or maybe he doesn't like poofs, like the rest of them here. I nearly got beaten up in the toilets for smiling at someone."

"No way!"

"Well, when I say smile, I also told him he had a nice arse. But I was just being friendly!"

"Be careful, will you. I don't think it's a good idea to try to pull straight men. And anyway, can't you think about something else than sex for one evening?"

"You're right, we're here for you. So go and get lucky!"
I follow James onto the dance floor, trying very hard not
to bump into people or collapse, until he finds an empty
spot. The music is loud and I don't recognise it, but I
dance, conscious of the people around us staring. I
catch a few men's eyes and can't help smiling. Then
they seem to come closer and closer, practically fighting
for my attention. I'm very, very drunk, but perfectly alert.
A tall, dark man, possibly Spanish or Asian, stands in
front of me, imitating my moves. I put my hands on his
waist and we dance together for a while, until his face
touches mine and we kiss passionately. His face is
smooth, and he smells of aftershave. I gently push him
away, turn around and repeat the same actions with
another guy, and then another. It's as if there was only
me and a hundred hungry men. After a while, ten,
maybe fifteen minutes later, James pulls me to the side.

"What are you doing?"

"Having fun! What are you doing?"

"Stopping you before you turn the dance floor into a
porn film set!"

"I don't know what you're talking about! I thought that's
what you wanted!"

"Of course not. I want you to come out of your shell,
yes, but not like that. These men were on you like
vultures on a corpse!"

"You can talk, Mr I get paid to have sex!"

"At least I know my limits. Come on, let's get you some
water. You've obviously had way too many drinks."

"You're just jealous!"

"Darling, trust me; there's nothing to be jealous of."

I am so, so embarrassed. I don't remember half of what happened, but I know it wasn't pretty. James had to practically drag me out of the club because I wouldn't go. I can't believe I snogged not one, not two, but at least four different men! I've never, ever done anything like that before. What if there were people I knew in that club? People from work, or a friend of my parents'? I'm grateful James looked after me; God knows what would have happened if he hadn't been around. I suppose if he hadn't been around, I wouldn't have been in that situation in the first place. But I shouldn't blame him, really. He was just trying to help. I had fun though. It was all that I resented in others, but somehow, I enjoyed it. And I honestly think I could do it again! With the right amount of alcohol, obviously. It was so nice to feel attractive and wanted. I get out of my flat, despite the hangover and go back to Oxford Street. I ignore the shoppers who bump into me, avoid the tourists taking pictures of window displays and that really annoying man with his speakerphone who goes on about Jesus and how to "be a winner, not a sinner." I wonder if he's employed by the local church, or if he's just a raving lunatic. I get a couple more skirts, some tight tops and do a speedy Christmas shopping run. Then I go home, pack my bags and head for my parents'. As usual, my mother hasn't put up any decorations and expects me and Jenny to do it, because she's convinced that we actually enjoy it. My dad is asleep and Jenny's out, so it's just me and her.

"How is Adam these days?" I refuse to tell her what happened, because it's all I'd hear about it for the whole week. She'd go on about how I probably pushed him away, what a great man he was and why on earth do I never make an effort in relationships.

"He's fine."

"I thought you might bring him. There is enough space in the house."

"He does have a family of his own, you know."

"Oh, of course. I expect you will be missing him lots, though. Feel free to use the phone."

"Where's Jenny?" I ask, trying to change the subject. It still hurts to think about him.

"Out with Jonathan."

"Who?"

"Jonathan, her boyfriend. Didn't I tell you?"

"No, you didn't. Who is he?" I ask, trying to sound interested, but I don't really want to know. No one can be good enough for her. And I'm slightly jealous.

"Remember that young man who came to my birthday dinner?"

"Him? Yes, I remember him. Anyway, I'm just going to unpack my stuff and…"

"He's rather handsome, isn't he? And very bright. He's a bit older than her, eighteen I think, but he is ever so polite. You two have done well for yourselves. Let's hope you keep it that way." She says tapping on my shoulder. "Would you like a cup of tea?"

There's no way I'm telling anyone about me and Adam. Ever. They'll all think I'm a failure and can't keep a man. Not that I really care, but I don't want to be compared to Jenny again. He was rather cute, that young guy. Jonathan and Jenny. That doesn't sound right, does it? Jonathan and Melanie sounds much better. I hope Adam's OK. I hope he's spending Christmas with his family and not just sitting in his messy flat, too miserable to go out or see anyone. James is right; if he were dead or in a really bad state I would have been told by now; but he could be suffering in silence, hiding in his dark bedroom, listening to his depressing music and carving horrible words into his skin and no one would know. Maybe I should call him. Maybe it'll show him that I can be his friend and that he's not alone. Or maybe he's getting better and I'll only bring back horrible memories and ruin his Christmas. Oh God, I don't know. I want so stuff myself with mince pies and Chocolate Roses.

"Guess who's coming for Christmas dinner?" My mother asks through my door. "Di and Patrick. The kids won't be around so I thought they'd like the company." Great. As if the whole thing wasn't stressful enough, now I'm going to have to be polite. "And Jonathan!" What? I nearly choke. "Did you hear me?"

"Yes. Why is he coming?"

"Because I invited him. His parents are going to a ball or something and he is part of this family now. Just like Adam." If hear his name one more time I'm going to pull my hair out. Although I shouldn't really complain; ever since she met him she's been much nicer to me. I wonder what I'm going to wear... I wasn't planning to make an effort, but since we'll have guests, maybe I should. I did bring a couple of nice outfits, just in case. "Darling, will you help me decide what to cook?" For Christ's sake. She does that every year. And every year I have to tell her there's no point asking me because I'll only make her buy vegetables and low fat cheese, but she still thinks she can't do it on her own. She's only been around for fifty odd years, after all. "Your phone's just beeped, dear. You must have left it downstairs. I wonder if it's Adam." Hair pulling session here I come.

"No, it won't be him." I say in a sigh as I open my front door .

"Why not?" She asks, clearly surprised.

"Because... he doesn't have a phone."

"Well he could have borrowed someone else's, just to see that you get here OK...."

"Mum! Please, can you stop talking about him for just five minutes?"

"Is there a problem? Has something happened?"

"No, nothing's happened. It's just... I miss him and it's hard when you remind me every two seconds that he's not here", I say in one breath.

"Of course darling. I'm sorry."

The message is from James. "Hey you little tart. How's the hangover?" I wish he were here. If he didn't have his own family I could invite him for Christmas dinner; mother wouldn't mind, since she's invited everyone else without consulting me. He'd certainly make the experience far more bearable. And I'm sure he'd rather be anywhere else than home; his lot sound like a real bunch of weirdos. His Mum lives with a man twenty years older than her and she's always denied they were together, although it's obvious since they have a one-bedroom house. His brother's in the army and his father hasn't spoken to him since he came out. So he's spending a few days at his sister's, who sounds like the only half decent person he's related to.

After I've unpacked, I go downstairs to watch TV. At this time of year it's always full of specials and repeats and repeats of specials, but it's an excuse not to talk. I bet James and his sister will spend Christmas Eve eating takeaways in front of Only Fools and Horses. I'd do anything to swap places with him. Christmas television was designed for dysfunctional families and we are definitely one of them.

"Ooh, the Vicar of Dibley!" My mother shouts and sits down next to me. Hasn't she got a cake to make or stockings to fill?

"Actually, I was going to flick through."

"Why? Don't you like The Vicar of Dibley?" I don't really want to tell her that I can't look at anyone bigger than Carol Vorderman without feeling nauseous, because she'd think I'm being mean.

"I've seen it too many times."

"Oh, I can never get bored of it. That Dawn French, isn't she marvellous?"

"Yeah. I prefer Jennifer Saunders."

"Really? Why?" Because she's thinner?

"Different sense of humour", I say as though I knew exactly what I was talking about.

"Oh, right. That Lenny Henry… why on earth did he feel the need to cheat on poor Dawn, it's beyond me." Because no one wants to shag ten tons of fat! She's already driving me mad and I've only been around her for a few hours. Soon she's going to offer me Quality Streets and force-feed me her apple crumble. Thankfully, the front door opens and Jenny comes in, but to my horror, with Jonathan! I wasn't told he'd be here! I look like shit!

"Hey Mel!" She gives me a hug. "Remember Jonathan?"

"Err, no, sorry", I say coolly, as if I were a socialite in front of a mere working class boy. "But nice to meet you." For all he knows, I could have hundreds of friends and meet new people everyday; how the hell am I expected to remember everyone?

"He was at Mum's birthday party."

"Oh yes, of course!"

"Of course you know who Jonathan is", my mother intervenes, "I only told you about him an hour ago!" Shit. I forgot about that. Now he probably thinks I'm completely stupid as well as ugly. Why did she have to open her mouth? "Are you staying for dinner, Jonathan dear?" What? Please make her stop!

"Nah thanks, I'm just picking up a CD." And off they go upstairs. Thank God.

"Isn't he lovely?"

"Yes. Adorable."

****

My mother's idea of Christmas decorations is a dozen Victorian-style balls bought from a pound shop, two strings of tinsel and every Santa, Angel and Rudolfs Jenny and I made at school since we were born. But thankfully this time, God knows how, I managed to persuade her not to buy chocolate decorations for the tree. I have a nice chat with Jenny, but as soon as we manage to put the plastic tree together, her phone rings and she leaves me to deal with the Victorian balls and paper Santas. I'm starting to feel jealous of her again. She's probably going to be out most nights this week and I'll be stuck at home with the specials. I could go out by myself. I wouldn't go to an actual place by myself, of course, but I could pretend I'm seeing a friend and just get on a bus and be driven to some random destinations for a couple of hours. I could even do that on Christmas Eve. I'd arrive a few minutes after everyone else, blaming my friend Joanna for making me stay out for one last drink. I don't know anyone called Joanna, but she could be a friend from work whose family lives in the area. What a brilliant idea.

Urgh. I've just that the most disturbing thought. What if Jonathan stays over on Christmas Eve? My room's right next to Jenny's and I would die if I heard her have sex. That's even worse than hearing my parents do it. I bet mother wouldn't even realise; she probably thinks Jenny's still a virgin and that he'd sleep on the floor. I wonder if it'll last. I wonder what he's like. And if he has an older brother. Or a twin. Oh God. What am I doing? I'm perving on my sister's boyfriend! Mother wasn't too happy when I mentioned Joanna.

"Can't you see her another day?"

"No, she's leaving on Boxing Day. She has to cover the phones."

"But surely if she's from work you can see her when you get back!"

"We… don't work together anymore."

"But you just told me she had to go back to your office to cover the phones!" Shit. My lying skills are really not so good these days.

"Not my office, another office. She's based in… Bristol", I say triumphantly, remembering the twisted ankle/hospital incident.

"Oh. Now I'm really confused. When I called your boss that time Jenny was in hospital, he told me you didn't have an office in Bristol." Jesus Christ! "Melanie, is there something you're not telling me? Are you seeing someone behind Adam's back?"

"What? No, of course not! And I didn't mean Bristol but Brighton. I always get them confused. We've just opened a call centre in Brighton." Please, please don't call them to check.

"Right. What time will you be back?" She says, clearly only half convinced.

"I don't know. What time does dinner start?"

"Well I was hoping you and Jenny would give me a hand preparing things, not just turn up to eat them."

"I'll do my best. What time are the guests coming?"

"Seven." Great. I'll help her in the afternoon, nip out at, say, five and come back at ten past seven. Perfect.

She drags me to the supermarket to get all the ingredients, insisting she has to make everything from scratch rather than buying it ready made. "That's part of the fun", she says. Well, not for me, thank you. She always leaves it to the last minute, which usually means there's hardly anything left in the shops. I don't personally care that much, but I don't understand why she can't do her Christmas shopping in October, like every other mum. She asks my opinion on every single thing she picks up, even though I keep telling her it makes no difference to me because I'll only eat the vegetables and condiments anyway. She's most definitely the reason why I hate shopping. She wanders into every single aisle, even the pets and DIY ones, for no reason whatsoever, walking so slowly one would think she were about a hundred years old. She reads the ingredients to everything (even eggs, for God's sake!), "just to make sure there's nothing toxic hidden inside". I don't know why she didn't ask Jenny to come instead. It's not fair. And then, once she's paid and I think the ordeal is over, she decides to stop at the cafeteria to have a cup of tea! Why not having one in the comfort of your own home, which is ten minutes away, I ask her. And I get told I have "no sense of community". Well, sorry for not considering myself to be part of a group of overweight teenage mothers with golden clown earrings!

"Look, it's Marianne Jones! Let's go and say hi", she says, and gets up.

"What about your tea? And the trolley?"

"Oh, right. Well, you stay here then." Good, because I'm really not in the mood to socialise. And I haven't a clue who Marianne bloody Jones is. But now I'm sitting on my own like an idiot and anyone could just come and start talking to me. After a minute or two, my mother comes back followed by another woman in a bright red suit, who I'm guessing is Marianne Jones.

"Melanie, you remember Marianne, don't you?"

"Err… yes, of course." I get up and shake her dry hand, trying hard to remember who the hell that woman is.

"And this is my son, Michael." A man probably my age and rather attractive, although wearing white tracksuit bottoms, appears behind her. He's tall, slim built, and has a goatee. Shit, I'm not dressed for this. You can't even do your food shopping without having to worry about bumping into people!

"Remember Michael, Melanie?" My mother says. "You used to be good friends at school. You had marble tournaments together." Oh, yes. Actually, I stole his marbles.

"Hi", he says quietly. He's clearly either shy or repulsed by me. Or maybe stealing his marbles scarred him for life.

"Hi", I reply, trying to sound casual.

"Michael lives in London too, now", my mother adds. "Maybe you two should meet up when you get back." She just can't help herself. She has to embarrass me all the bloody time, even in front of people I haven't seen for fifteen years.

"Sure", I say, not looking at him for fear of seeing a "Yeah, right!" look on his face.

"Mum, I really have to go or I'm going to miss the match", Michael says. "Nice seeing you again, Melanie." I knew it. He thinks I'm repulsive.

"Well, wasn't it nice?" My mother says as they walk off.

"Yes. Enlightening conversation."

"Don't be so sarcastic. He's a lovely lad, he is."

"How would you know? You think everyone's lovely."

"Is it a crime to see the good in people?"

"No, mother. I just don't think there was much to see in a thirty-second exchange of small talk."

"Melanie, you are so nonchalant. No wonder it took you so long to find a boyfriend."

****

The one thing I like about Christmas is the snow. It doesn't snow often, but this year we're lucky enough to get a few inches of it. It makes everything look so quaint and small. I used to make snowmen with Jenny when we were little. Come to think of it, we only stopped four years ago, when she decided she was "grown up" and it wasn't cool enough. Personally, I still like them. But I'm too embarrassed to make them by myself. On the other hand, I hate snowballs. I've learnt never to walk past children who play with snow, because they always end up getting me. Once, when I was ten, someone put a stone inside a snowball and it hit me on the forehead. I still have the scar.

My mother made me get up at nine this morning, because she decided the house had to be clean and tidy by lunchtime. Thing is, it's always clean and tidy, because she spends nearly two hours every day hoovering and doing the surfaces. She made me hoover my room, which was completely pointless because a) I've only been in it for three days and b), I'm not going to let anyone in it tonight. Then she asked me to finish the cake, which I refused to do for reasons she still doesn't get, but that obviously I couldn't explain to her; so she accused me of being lazy and unhelpful. So I sulked and she sulked, and we spent about two hours not talking to each other. I stayed in my room and watched the snow. When I came down she'd nearly finished all the preparations, so all I had to do was lay the table. Then I got ready to go out – I figured since everyone will be here when I get back, I won't have time to get changed – and now I'm on my bus ride. It's actually quite nice to be driven to new places and not having a clue where you'll end up. Except that it's dark and still snowing, so I can't see much outside apart from hundreds of Christmas lights. Still, it'll be worth it in the end. The bus is quiet; the only people upstairs with me are a Chinese couple, an old woman and a drunk man who keeps talking to himself. I wonder if they're going somewhere, or if, like me, they're just killing time. I wonder if the old woman has a family to go to and if the drunk man has a place to live, or if he's just going to spend Christmas going on bus rides to keep warm. I feel sad. I don't understand how some people, like my mother, are so worried about how much food to buy for dinner and how many people to cook for, when some others will have to survive on bread crumbs, if they're lucky. There should be vans going around houses after dinner tonight, collecting all the leftovers and giving them to the homeless. Maybe I should write to the council. Or the Minister of Homelessness, or whatever he/she is called these days. Hang on. What is going on outside? We haven't moved for about half an hour. There's traffic everywhere. Right, I've been on this bus for about an hour, it's a quarter to six, if I get off at the next stop, which hopefully we should reach quite soon, I should be OK. Thankfully, shortly after, we start moving... but only very, very slowly. Twenty minutes later and we haven't got very far. I walk down, nearly falling over the slippery stairs and ask the driver where the next stop is.

"Usually, we'd get there in two minutes from here. But given the traffic, it's going to take at least another half hour." Shit. "Where are you going?" Why does he need to know?

"Meopham."

"Meopham? But that's in the opposite direction!"

"I know. Can you let me out soon?"

"There wouldn't be much point, really. You won't find a bus stop to Meopham around here."

"Well how long will it take to walk to the next bus stop?"

"Not long, I suppose. But it is snowing quite heavily."

"That's fine." He lets me out, so I cross the road, and following his directions, make my way to the bus stop. It is snowing really heavily and it's absolutely freezing. I brought my umbrella, but as it's also windy, it's not much use. I'm going to look like such a mess when I get home. I walk with great difficulty for a good ten minutes, until I find the petrol station where the bus stop is. I look at the timetable and to my horror, it looks like I've just missed a bus and the next one isn't coming for another half hour! I'm going to be in so much trouble! I go to petrol station to buy some coffee and get warm and as I wait for it to come out of the machine, I see a sign for a taxi company. Great idea! I call the number, feeling relieved, but then, I nearly die: fifty pounds to get back to my house!

"It's Christmas Eve", the man at the other end says. "It's more expensive." So I have to choose between getting told off in front of my aunt, uncle and sister's boyfriend, i.e., being totally humiliated, or not being able to eat and drink for at least a week. I choose the latter. But the closer we get to home, the more I realise that I'm going to get told off anyway and I should have kept my money for a night out with James to recover. At half seven, I'm on the doorstep. I pull myself together, reapply some make up and brush my hair, take a deep breath and open the front door. My mother appears straight away, carrying a tray of mini pizzas and vol au vents.

"Where on earth have you been? And what are you wearing?"

"Sorry, I left really early but there were no buses. I had to get a cab", I say, hoping she'll offer me some of the money back. But she just shakes her head and points at the lounge.

"Go and say hello to everyone. You could have taken your phone with you. I called you about twenty times."

"Sorry." I walk to the lounge, where everyone is sat, drinking and eating appetisers.

"Melanie, how nice of you to join us!" Patrick says with the usual smug look on his face. Then he looks me up and down. "Wow. I didn't know you had legs!" Funnily enough, it was much more flattering when said by someone in my office. Pervert.

"Mel, you look gorgeous!" Jenny says, her mouth wide open.

"It's very… different", my father says, clearly shocked.

"Hi Melanie", Di simply says and gives me a hug.

"Hi Jonathan!" I say in my friendliest voice and shake his hand.

"Hi…ya."

"You shouldn't go out dressed like that, especially at this time of the year", my mother says. "You could get yourself into trouble."

"I'm fine. I do it all the time in London", I reply as coolly as I can.

"Since when?" She says, obviously unimpressed. I shrug, and help myself to a whiskey.

"I think it's great!" Patrick says, winking at me. Urgh.

"Well we'll talk about it later", mother says. "Let's have dinner."

I'd planned to stuff myself with fruit before coming back, so I wouldn't be tempted by anything, but with all the bus drama I completely forgot. I've no idea what any of the food is (by the time everyone had got to the dinner table I'd already had three whiskeys), but it looks delicious. I wish mother wasn't such a good cook, it's absolute torture. I have to remind myself that Jonathan's here, otherwise I'd probably lick everyone's plates. But just as everything was going surprisingly well, Patrick opens his mouth again.

"By the way, Melanie, where's... what's his name, Alan?" I take a deep breath.

"Adam."

"Adam! That's right. How is Adam?"

"He's fine."

"Not here?"

"Clearly not", I reply sarcastically.

"Well, where is he then?" For fuck's sake.

"With his family."

"Oh. Not very gentleman-like to abandon his girlfriend at Christmas, is it?"

"Patrick!" Di finally says. She hadn't opened her mouth since we said hi.

"I'm just being concerned for our Melanie." If I were in front of him I'd give him a good kick.

"I'm sure she's doing just fine", Di says grumpily. Thankfully, the subject moves on to Jonathan's degree and I listen eagerly, although not being quite sure exactly what he's talking about. He is really, really good looking, despite the fact that he's wearing what looks like a jumper knitted by a blind person on drugs.

"What is it you said your degree was?" I ask him.

"Molecular Biology." Oh God. I hate biology.

"Really? That's great. So… fascinating."

"It's early days, but so far it's been good."

"Since when do you like sciences?" My mother intervenes." She used to hate it at school, it was such an ordeal trying to make her do her homework", she adds to Jonathan.

"Well I like it now", I reply dryly, but still trying to smile. "A…ny…way. What would you like to do with your Moliculor degree?" For some reason, everyone laughs.

"Molecular, Melanie!"

"What? That's what I said!"

"Research, probably", Jonathan replies.

"Wow. Not just a pretty face!" I say, nodding. And then Patrick laughs, Jenny gives me a horrified look and I realise what I've just said. "I mean… it's nice to meet people who have half a brain these days, especially when they're so young…. Not that you're very young, obviously, but younger than me… Not that I'm more intelligent than you because I'm older, obviously…" Oh God, someone please stop me. Why did I have to drink so much whiskey? "Anyway, Di, how's things?" She stops eating, stares at her plate and bursts into tears. Mother gives me a disapproving look and shakes her head. "What?" I whisper. I glance at Patrick, who's sitting still and clearly uncomfortable. Di gets up and runs to the loo.

"We're getting divorced", Patrick says after a long silence. Divorced? I can't say I'm surprised. About bloody time, actually.

"Sorry. I didn't know."

"You would have if you hadn't arrived two hours late!" mother shouts.

"Well I'm sorry but it hadn't occurred to me that this would be the kind of conversation to have before a Christmas dinner!"

"I would have told you before everyone got here", she replies quietly. "I found out this afternoon."

"I'm sorry, but shouldn't you be comforting her?" I ask Patrick angrily. "After all, it's quite obvious why this has happened, isn't it? She finally saw sense! How many women did you have to sleep with before she realised?"

"I didn't. She's the one who had an affair."

"I'm sorry Jonathan", my mother says after a long silence. "She's not usually like this."

****

It was an easy mistake to make. At least, Jonathan thought I was cool. Well, hilarious is the word he apparently used, but it's the same thing, isn't it? And anyway, it's very unlikely that I'll be seeing Patrick ever again, so who cares? Jenny wasn't too pleased about me coming on to her boyfriend, but I think she's forgiven me now. I've invited them over to make up for it and promised her I wouldn't get drunk in front of them. James laughed his head off when I told him. I'm considering spending next Christmas with him and his sister; it seems like a much safer option. But now that I'm back in London, I find myself missing home. It was nice not to have to worry about using electricity and buying food. Now I'm going to have to work for at least two weeks before I can start spending anything. James offered to lend me some money, but I hate being in debt. He only came back on January 2nd, so I spent New Year's Eve on my own, watching videos and trying to ignore all the drunk people celebrating outside.

Secretly, I kind of wish I'd been one of them. I used to spend New Year's Eve with Naomi, but I didn't dare ask her; I figured she'd be stuck at home with George, not able to drink anything. Still, a bit of company would have been nice. I felt like a real saddo.

After a few days of hermitage, I give in to James's nagging and we go to a club call The Scala in King's Cross, on Andrew's recommendation. It's a rather nice place, spread out on three floors, with varied music and lots of attractive men, although it's hard to tell which ones are straight and which ones aren't. I felt very self-conscious at first; I was worried about how much weight I'd put on over Christmas. But James, bless him, managed to sort me out quickly, like he usually does.

We make a bet of finding as many straight/gay men as possible and snogging them, but after three hours of heavy drinking, we both lose count. I wasn't supposed to stay late because I have to work in the morning, but I end up getting home at five, oversleeping, and arriving at the office late and still half drunk. Thankfully Phil is off sick, so I don't get told off; but I do mix up a few feedback forms and when I get home, I realise I haven't turned my computer off and as I'm not working tomorrow (I wanted to do a full week but three other supervisors had already booked Monday), anyone could look in my files and get confidential stuff out. But if anyone says anything, I can always blame my pc for not shutting down properly. Or the cleaner. At half eight, just as I was dozing off, the phone rings and I nearly die: it's

Michael! Apparently his mother bumped into my mother again and she gave her my phone number because Michael wanted to meet up... so we're going for a drink tomorrow night. I can't quite believe it. Why would he like me since he's only seen me with practically no makeup on and baggy trousers? Maybe my mother's behind it. Maybe she's paid him to ask me out for one reason or another. I should have asked him. I mean, why on earth would he want to hang out with someone he hasn't seen properly for a dozen years? It's quite exciting, though. I decide to wear my knee-length suede like cream skirt, a short-sleeved black top, and a satin thong, just for confidence. We meet outside a small pub on Wardour Street and at first I don't recognise him: his hair is shorter, he's clearly just shaved and most shocking of all, he's wearing a suit!

Like a true gentleman, he lets me in first, buys me a drink and pulls out a chair for me. He asks me about my job, where I live and what I like to do. Then I ask him the same and that's when it all goes wrong. He works for Chelsea United, lives in Chelsea and during his spare time, he watches football, collects football kits and is even writing a book about one of Chelsea's players, God knows his name; I'd stopped listening by that point. But the thing is, the more I drink, the more I want to kiss him. After nearly two hours of ranting, I decide to make a move.

"Enough about football, Mike", I say, bringing my lips close to his. At first he moves slightly backwards, but quickly gives in to passion.

"Do you want to come back to mine? It wouldn't take long in a cab", he says shortly after.

"Can't we stay here for now?" I don't give him time to reply, I grab his face and kiss him again. But he puts his hand on my lips.

"We could do this in my flat. It's… cosier." Suddenly I feel nervous. Trapped, like I've started something I can't stop. Like I have to go all the way. But I don't want to. I burst into tears. "What's wrong? What did I say?"

"I… I don't… want to sleep… with you!" I say between sobs.

"Hey, don't worry about it. That's cool."

"Why do you want to sleep with me anyway? I'm ugly and fat and repulsive!"

"What are you talking about?"

"It's because of my mother, isn't it? She told you I was a failure and you just feel sorry for me!"

"Melanie, I honestly don't know what…"

"Why would you want me when you could have her?" I say pointing at a tall blonde at the bar.

"Come on, let's get you home." He gets up and grabs my arm.

"No! I don't want to!"

"Is everything alright?" says a big guy with a beard behind Michael.

"What do you think?" I shout.

"Yes, we're fine, thanks. Melanie, I'm not going to do anything. I just want to help you get home alright."

"Why? It's pointless. I'm pathetic!"

"Of course you're not pathetic. You've just had a few too many drinks." He walks me to the tube and waits with me for a train.

"Thank you", I say as one pulls in.

"Will you be OK getting home?"

"I'll be fine. Sorry I ruined your evening."

"Don't worry. Text me when you get home so I know you're alright."

I get home, text him, throw myself into bed and bury my head under my pillow, swearing never to leave my room ever again.

****

Shit. I was late for work again. Phil wasn't happy. I told him I was recovering from food poisoning, but the smokey smell in my hair and the makeup all over my face might have been a giveaway. Plus he told me off for the feedback sheets and my computer being left on. I didn't have the strength to argue, or lie. Michael texted me, to ask if I was feeling better. I don't know what to do; I'm so embarrassed about what happened, but he was so nice about it. It could have all gone wrong. Well, worse, anyway. I hope he doesn't want to see me again, though. I don't think I could handle it. But what if he tells his mum what happened and she tells mine? I couldn't deal with her being on my case as well. Maybe I should see him again, just to show him I'm perfectly normal. But if I ask him out he'll probably think I'm clingy! Best to leave it in his hands, I suppose. I reply that I'm fine, sorry again, etc and as soon as I send the message, Phil is on my case again.

"Melanie, can you please wait for your break before using your mobile phone?" He talks to me like I'm a kid today. I'm a supervisor, for Christ's sake, surely I'm allowed to use my phone to send a stupid text message!

He's just jealous because he doesn't have a life. "And the kitchen is a bit messy", he adds. Fuck off!

I get back home to a tearful message from Naomi. I hadn't heard from her since we bumped into each other that afternoon. Seems that things aren't going so well with George. I spend over half an hour trying to calm her down and I end up going to her flat the next evening.

"It's since I told him I was pregnant", she says blowing her nose. "I don't think he fancies me anymore."

"But you don't look any different, apart from having a few more pounds on. You're still stunning."

"Well, tell him that! He's freaked out, that's what it is. He doesn't like the fact that there's a human life inside my body." To be honest, I don't blame him.

"But I thought you said he was OK about it?"

"That's what I thought too. But he was just playing for time. In a few months time, there'll be a baby and I'm going to be all alone to raise it!"

"Of course you won't. Your parents will be there. And I'll be there too." She stops sobbing and looks up.

"Really? You'll help me?"

"Well… Yes. As much as I can."

"Oh, thank you so much, Mel! I knew I could count on you. You don't know how much this means to me!" Oh gosh. I only meant I'd be on the other end of the phone! "I know you don't really like babies, but maybe this one will make you change your mind!" she says pointing at her belly. Never in a million years!

"So… what are you going to do about George?"

She sighs. "End it and move in with my parents, I suppose. I don't know why he hasn't dumped me yet. Bloody coward."

"Where is he tonight?"

"With his mates, as usual. Oh Mel, what have I done?" She bursts into tears again.

"Don't worry, it'll all be OK in the end", I say stroking her hair.

"You think so?" I bite my lip.

"Y...yeah. Of course."

"I'm so sorry. I haven't even asked you how you were. And how's it going with Adam?"

"We've split up."

"Really? I'm sorry."

"Don't be. It was for the best. I'm doing fine."

"So it's just like the old times, then. You and me."

"I... suppose, yes." I hope she doesn't expect me to stay in with her on Saturday nights to talk about sour nipples and smelly nappies.

****

"Take a seat, Miss Stevenson", a tall, grey-haired man says as he opens the door to a small, yellow-painted office where John, Chrissie and two other people are sitting. They all have pens and notepads and as I sit down, they all smile awkwardly. "I'm Doctor Johnson and these are my colleagues, Doctor Brown and Doctor Barnett. And you obviously know John and Chrissie. So, we are here today because you wish to discuss your diagnosis. Is that right ? " We talk about my past and current issues, my progress, my symptoms and after forty minutes, he finally breaks it to me.

"Borderline Personality Disorder."

At the end of my appointment, I go to the library and borrow a medical book.

Borderline Personality Disorder: A pervasive pattern of instability of interpersonal relationships, self-image and affects and marked impulsivity beginning by early adulthood and present in a variety of contexts, as indicated by five (or more) of the following:

Frantic efforts to avoid real or imagined abandonment.

A pattern of unstable and intense interpersonal relationships characterised by alternating between extremes of idealisation and devaluation.

Identity disturbance: markedly and persistently unstable self-image or sense of self.

Impulsivity in at least two areas that are potentially self-damaging (e.g., spending, sex, substance abuse, reckless driving, binge eating).

Recurrent suicidal behaviour, gestures, or threats, or self-mutilating behaviour.

Affective instability due to a marked reactivity of mood (e.g., intense episodic dysphoria, irritability, or anxiety usually lasting a few hours and only rarely more than a few days).

Chronic feelings of emptiness.

Inappropriate, intense anger or difficulty controlling anger (e.g., frequent displays of temper, constant anger, recurrent physical fights).

Transient, stress-related paranoid ideation or severe dissociative symptoms.

I read on, tears rolling down my face. It's all there. It's all me. There's an explanation for everything I do or feel. I have a disorder. I don't know if I should feel better now, or worse. At least I don't suffer from some obscure illness that no one's ever come across. And now, whatever I do wrong, I can say, "It's not my fault, it's my disorder." But I've been put into a box and I fit in it perfectly. I walk down to the corner shop and buy three boxes of Hob Nobs and a bottle of wine. Half way down the second box, I hear the front door open, steps walking up and the sound of a key in James's door. I wipe the crumbs off my face and head for his room.

"I have a borderline personality disorder!", I say, half sobbing, as he opens the door.

"You have a what?"

"Borderline personality disorder!"

"Oh. Is that bad?"

"Of course it's bad!"

"Oh", he repeats and then goes silent.

"I'm a freak!"

"Well, we both knew that already darling." He laughs, then stops when he sees the angry look on my face.

"Sorry. Look, at the end of the day, you're still the same person you were yesterday. It's just a word."

"Three words, actually." We look at each other and giggle.

"So what do these three words actually mean?"

"They mean I'm a paranoid-impulsive-moody-suicidal overeater."

"Wow. Sounds impressive."

"Or that I belong in a circus, more like."

"Well, I always thought your talents were wasted in Market Research. Anyway, I've had a shit day too; fancy getting plastered?"

"I shouldn't ; I have to work tomorrow. "

"So what ? A few drinks won't kill you. And it's not the first time you'll go to work with a hangover. "

"Exactly. I could get into trouble."

"Of course you won't. They can't sack you for a hangover." I sigh. I really feel like getting drunk, actually. And after all, according to that medical book that's what people with Borderline Personality Disorder do.

"Alright then. As long as we don't stay out too late."

     I get back home at midnight, got to bed at twenty past and go to sleep at around half one… and wake up with another painful hangover. I manage to drag myself to the office on time, and everything seems to go surprisingly well, until Phil tells me at half past three that I've been giving everyone a survey they completed last week.

"In my defence, why didn't any of them notice?"

"You're not in a position to be asking questions, Melanie. It was your responsibility to give them the right survey. "

"I do realise that, but... "

"I'm very concerned with the recent level of your work. You turn up late, you make mistakes you would never have made a few months ago... Are you still happy here? " I've never been happy here, I want to say.

"Well... Yes. "

"Then I want to see some improvement. I'm giving you a warning for today's events. " A warning ? I've never had a warning before! Oh God. I've screwed up big time. I knew he didn't like me! It's not fair. Now that things were finally starting to be good, he has to spoil it!

Chapter 8

I have to pull myself together. No more going out on school nights, no more drinking. Apart from tonight, as Andrew has invited me and James to his birthday party. And I'm not working tomorrow anyway, so no risk of another warning yet. I thought I'd only be surrounded by gay men, so I didn't make too much effort – and I didn't have any clean tights – so I'm wearing a long denim skirt and white shirt, but it turns out Andrew has four rather attractive straight male friends, three of whom are apparently single. James supplies me with double vodkas and after a few shots, having managed to pull my skirt up a little without getting noticed, I decide to introduce myself.

" Hi! I'm... Melanie", I say trying as much as possible to smile.

" Nice to meet you again, Melanie ", the blond guy says and the other three giggle.

"Again? "

"Andrew introduced us about an hour ago. " Huh. I don't remember that. I didn't think I was that drunk!

" Oh yes! Of... course ! Sorry, terrible memory. I did think you looked familiar! "

" No worries. I'm Crispin."

" Hi Cripsin ! Err... Crispin, sorry." I turn to his friends, only to realise they've disappeared. "Oh. "

"I think they went to get another drink. "

" It's the skirt, isn't it ", I say sadly.

" Sorry? "

I head for the bar, where James is writing his phone number on a matchbox.

" Have you pulled? " I ask, already knowing the answer.

" Too right. Gorgeous lawyer. "

" Is my skirt too long? "

"Darling, for the ten millionth time, your skirt is fine! Your top if fine, your hair's perfect, stop freaking out!" He walks off, so I sit myself on a stool at the counter and order another vodka.

"Are you OK? " Says Crispin, who appears shortly after.

"Yes. I just needed a drink. "

" Can I buy you the next one? " Oh. Maybe James is right after all!

"Sure", I say and down my vodka. After finishing the one he bought me, I insist on getting him one in return; and after a couple more rounds and a lot of small talk, I hear myself say: "Do you want to come back to mine?" But he stays silent.

"I get it", I say my eyes watering. "The only thing you could possibly like about me is my legs and you can't even see them."

"What? It's got nothing to do with your legs, or the rest of you. It's just that I have to work tomorrow."

"So you don't think I'm ugly?"

"Of course not", he says, although there's a strange look on his face.

"But do you think I'm attractive?" He laughs.

"Yes, you are very attractive. You shouldn't be so insecure."

"Then come home with me", I say grabbing his hand. I don't want to sleep with him... I don't even want to kiss him. But I need to feel wanted.

I make us a drink, put some music on, turn the light off and let him take off my clothes. He does whatever he has to do, which seems to take an awfully long time and when he's finally done, he offers to touch me, so I turn him away. He falls asleep and I stare at the clock until the next morning when he gets up and leaves, unaware that I'm awake and watching him. I get out of bed at lunchtime, feeling nauseous and dirty and have a long bath. I wonder if he did find me attractive, or if he just saw me as an easy shag. I should have asked him this morning.

****

The next few weeks are totally awful at work. Phil is constantly on my case and even though nothing disastrous happens, I know that secretly, he's waiting for the smallest faux-pas to get rid of me. I manage to stay sober quite well, though; or rather, not to get so drunk that I fuck up everything the next day. But on February 1st, comes the annual Corporate Evening at Dover Street Wine Bar, where the company takes its two biggest clients out on a drinking binge to thank them for giving us their money. I never had to go until now, although it was always strongly recommended by Phil, but this year, as I'm a supervisor, I don't have a choice. As it's a "Corporate Event" I have to look smart, which means, by Phil's standards, no minis, so I'm wearing a long black velvety dress which I just got from Dorothy Perkins, but, frankly, it looks more like something to wear at a cocktail party than at a wine bar. But everyone complements me on it, even Phil. Unfortunately, the corporate world, as I feared, is a rather dull one and full of arrogant overweight middle-aged men and their whorish secretaries, so I spend most of the evening by the bar, refilling my drink and pretending to text people when Phil isn't looking.

"You look rather bored", says a man probably in his thirties, tall and clean shaved. "I'm Eric Radcliff."

"Melanie Stevenson", I reply, as if I were a multimillionaire entrepreneur and my name would mean something to him.

"Nice to meet you, Melanie", he says shaking my hand. "So, what do you do when you don't attend magnificent corporate events?" He asks with a sarcastic tone.

"I'm a supervisor. Rather boring. What about you?" I ask trying to sound interested.

"Something rather boring too, unfortunately. So what do you do in your free time, what keeps you going?" I have to think hard. I don't actually do anything apart from going out and getting drunk. It's quite sad, actually.

"Socialise... Drink too much... the usual", I throw in casually.

"Ah! Now that's interesting." Is it? "And where do you socialise?" Oh God. Does he expect me to say the Ritz or something?

"You wouldn't know my bars."

"Oh, you'd be surprised! I know a wide range of eclectic places."

"OK then. First Out, The Observatory, G.A.Y?" He frowns. Thought so.

"No, I'm afraid, doesn't mean anything to me. Tell you what… Why don't we finish this drink and then you can take me to one of them?" I laugh.

"I… don't think that would be a good idea."

"Why not? I'm always looking for new places to hang out."

"I don't think they'd be your style."

"So what do you think would be my style?" He asks, clearly offended. Oh what the hell.

"OK then. But don't blame me if you hate it."

"I promise I won't."

We jump in a cab and head for The Observatory, the only place I thought he might actually be allowed in. With all the excitement, I'd forgotten what I was wearing and as we walk in, a few people give us amused looks.

"Is this… a gay bar?" He asks, half laughing.

"Yeah. I did try to warn you!"

"Well, it's OK, I don't mind. Let's get some drinks in." He rushes to the bar, buys me a drink and we sit at an empty table. "So…" He says, hesitantly. "Are you… gay?"

"No, not at all! I just like it here."

"Oh, good. I mean…" I let him struggle for a few seconds, amused. He looks quite attractive in his suit… a bit like Colin Firth in Bridget Jones's Diary. I wonder if he likes me. I down my drink and giggle.

"Don't worry, I know what you mean. Another one?" I ask, pointing to his glass.

"Sure."

A couple of hours later, we're in my house drinking shots and slagging off everyone we work with. But as I pour myself another vodka, he takes out of his wallet a little bag with white powder in it.

"Want some?" He says shaking the bag.

"What is it?" He laughs. "No, seriously, what is it?"

"It's coke", he says casually. My heart nearly stops.

"Coke? You brought drugs into my house?"

"It's alright, no need to shout. I'll put it back in my bag if you want. Look, gone now", he says patronisingly. I'm really thrown.

"I can't believe you brought drugs here! You could have got me into trouble with the police!" I shout, shaking.

"Nothing's going happen unless you don't chill out!" He says angrily. "Let's just forget about it, OK? It's no big deal."

"Well, yes it is a big deal to me, actually. Please go."

"What?"

"I said, go!" If I weren't so drunk, I'd probably be frightened to death. But right now, I'm just extremely pissed off. He gets up, grabs his jacket, opens my door and storms out.

"Bitch!"

****

Everyone knows. Or at least, they think they know. They're all giving me looks and whispering when I walk past. It's driving me insane. OK, I was stupid enough to "befriend" a client, but what's the big deal?

And why do they assume that we slept together? It's pathetic. Phil comes in at lunchtime, locks himself in his office for half an hour, then calls me in.

"You probably know why you're here", he says dryly.

"Nothing happened. We just went for a drink somewhere else, and that's it."

"That's not what I've heard."

"Well you've heard wrong", I say, trying hard to keep calm.

"That's not the point. Your attitude was extremely unprofessional. And it's made the company look unprofessional. It's put us in a very uncomfortable position. What kind of image do you think that portrayed?" Why is he acting like this?

"It was just a drink!"

"You were supposed to entertain all the clients, not just the one you fancied!" That is so out of order.

"I didn't fancy him, I was just being nice. Not that it's any of your business…"

"Oh, it is my business when the company's reputation is involved!" He shouts and makes me jump.

"I've told you before, Melanie. What you do in your own time is up to you, but if it affects your work, then I'm going to get involved. And this time it's gone too far. I'm sorry but you're forcing me to let you go." It takes me a while to realise what he's just said.

"What?"

"I will give you a good reference, because until recently, you were an amazing employee. I know you have issues, but I have to put the welfare of the company first."

"You're sacking me?"

"I'm sorry. You don't give me the choice. I did warn you."

I walk out of his office, head down. I pick up my jacket and my bag and leave, everyone staring at me. Why did he do that? I thought he was on my side! I spend the next few days hiding under my covers, crying and wishing I'd never been born. I knew it would happen. I'm a failure. An ugly, useless, failure. After three days, I give in to James's endless calls and knocks and tell him. As usual, he tries to show me the positive side of it, but frankly, I fail to see it. The company has given me a month's redundancy cheque, but a month goes quickly and if I don't find something else soon, I could end up homeless. He takes the next day off and drags me to the Job Centre, where apparently someone will help me find a job and give me some money whilst I'm unemployed. After queuing for over half an hour, the receptionist hands me three different forms, all about twenty pages each, which I have to fill out and return before I can see anyone else.

"What should I put under skills? I don't think I have any. And how am I supposed to look for work when I don't know what I want to do?"

"Just write anything. You don't really want them to give you a job, you just want the money."

"Really? Why?"

"Because they'll offer you shit like cleaning lady or care assistant or something."

"So how am I supposed to find work?"

"Well, knowing what you want to do would help. How about working for another Market Research company?"

"I'd rather not."

"I could ask at Virgin, they might have something."

"What, stacking shelves?" I laugh, and he raises his eyebrows. "Sorry. I just meant, I don't think I could do it." He smiles nonchalantly and flicks through the TV guide. "You know your escort thing", I say after a short silence. He looks up, dubious.

"Y...Yes?"

"Do you have to sleep with them every time?"

"I thought you weren't going to give me a hard time about it anymore?"

"I'm not! I'm just... interested."

"Well, yes, I do. But I don't escort mingers. Why are you interested?"

"No reason. Just... you know, wondering."

"Are you thinking of joining in?"

"No! Not if... I have to sleep with them. I just thought if I could keep them company for a couple of hours, it wouldn't do me any harm."

"True, but unfortunately it doesn't work like that with men. Unless..." He scratches his head, looks at me and nod.

"Unless what?"

"Unless you escort women." I giggle.

"What?"

"I'm serious. You could be a lesbian escort."

"For the millionth time, I'm not a fucking dyke!"

"Yeah, but they don't need to know that. See, most men are, as we all know, only interested in one thing,

252

regardless of whether they're straight or gay. But women, they want comfort, kindness, company. If you tell them you don't want sex, they won't care. Just take them to the cinema or something and they'll be happy.

"Are you serious?"

"Of course. I have a girlfriend who does it."

"And she's straight?"

"Well, no, but as I said, no one would know. It's a brilliant plan, if you ask me. And you wouldn't have to do it a lot, just a few times until you find a proper job. What do you think?"

****

Laura, 20, very feminine & attractive, offers her services to any woman, anywhere, any time.

"How does that look?"

"I think services implies there'll be sex involved. And any woman sounds weird."

"OK, what about this then?"

Laura, 20, very feminine & attractive, offers her company to women exclusively, anywhere, any time.

"Err, London only, please. I don't want to end up in Wales or something.

"OK... and what about prices? I don't think we should give it out in the ad, but we could say competitive.

"You know best."

"Check this out."

Laura, 20, very feminine & attractive, offers her company to women exclusively. London & surroundings, competitive prices.

"They'll pay for your travel expenses anyway."

"How much do you think I'm worth?" I say, getting quite excited.

"Probably about fifty an hour."

"Fifty? That much?"

"You could make much more once you've had a bit of experience."

"Really? Gosh. That's about what I used to get in a day. Remind me why I have to call myself Laura and be two years younger?"

"You need a stage name. It's a way to stay anonymous and to distance yourself from it. Same thing for the age. So it's not really you doing it, it's your character."

"Is that how you cope with the sex then?"

"Pretty much. So if I do something really naughty, I don't blame myself, I blame Fred."

"Fred? Is that what they call you?" I laugh.

"It's a perfectly acceptable name."

"I'm still not sure about it. What if something goes wrong?"

"What could go wrong? It'll only be for a few hours and then you don't have to see them ever again."

Although I'm nervous, I'm also quite excited. I'm going to get paid to go out with someone!

Two days later, as I come out of the Job Centre, my phone rings. I don't recognise the number so I send it to my voicemail, but it rings again shortly after. I pick up, just in case it's Phil offering me my job back.

"Is that Laura?" A faint voice asks.

"Sorry?"

"I was... looking for Laura." Shit! It worked! Oh God, what should I say? I clear my throat.

"Yes, hello there", I say as assured as I can.

"Hi. I saw your advert and I was wondering if you would be free on Friday night?" Damn. I was planning to go to G.A.Y with James and Andrew.

"Y... Yes, I am. What... would you like to do?"

"We could go for a drink somewhere, and maybe have dinner?" Huh. I was hoping we'd go to the cinema, so I wouldn't have to talk too much.

"Y... Yes, sure. What time would you like to meet?"

"Is seven OK for you?"

"Yes, that's fine", I say trying to find a pen in my bag. Whereabouts?" She gives me the address of a pub in Lewisham, probably my least favourite area in London and she describes herself as small, with short dark hair, and will be wearing a long brown coat.

Before I go to meet her, James briefs me on the dos and don'ts of escorting. "Do try to be nice and polite, even if she's a complete minger. Remember she's paying you and she expects a good service. But don't, under any circumstances, go back to her house, even if it's to show you her three cats."

"How do you know she has three cats?"

"She's a lesbian, isn't she? Chances are she's vegetarian, too. And make sure she knows she can't get into your pants."

"But what if she asks? I can't tell her she's not my type, right?"

"Definitely not. Say you're already spoken for. Or that it always takes you a few dates before you sleep with a client, then you're guaranteed another couple of evenings with her. And when she gets too desperate, just dump her and take on someone else."

"That sounds a bit harsh."

"It's business, darling. Don't wear too much makeup and no skirt, OK? You want to look credible. Act confident. And remember, she's supposed to buy you all the drinks."

So there I am, in denim jeans, white t-shirt and black cardigan, at the Rising Sun in Lewisham. I get there early, to make sure I'd spot her when she walks in and can't decide whether I really want to go through with it or run away. Half an hour and two glasses of wine later, a short woman with a long brown coat walks in, head down, and rushes to the toilets. Oh God, this is it. My heart is racing and my hands are shaking. I can't go now, I've come all this way and sat in this dodgy pub by myself to do business, and business I'm going to do. She comes out of the loo shortly after, buys a Bacardi Breezier, and sits a few tables away from mine. I count until ten and get up, then realise that I don't even know her name. If it's not her, I'm going to look like a complete prick! Money. Think about the money.

"Hi... I'm Laura." She gets up and shakes my hand.

"Hi... I'm Stephanie." OK, so it seems I've got the right person. Good start. "Would you like a drink?" I'm about to say I'll get it, when James's words pop back into my head. "Confidence. She's supposed to pay for your drinks."

"House white wine, please." This is so weird. I've never had a woman buy me a drink before. At least I asked for a cheap wine. Come to think of it, maybe I could have asked for a nicer one. She's got the money, after all. She's surprisingly pretty; although she's probably in her mid thirties, she has a very young face, with little green eyes and freckles. And she seems even more scared than I am.

"So", I say in my friendliest voice. "What do you do?"

"I'm a teacher", she replies, not really looking at me.

"What do you teach?"

"History." How boring.

"History! That's interesting", I say joyfully, and take a long sip of wine.

"It's… OK", she replies, half smiling. Then, there's silence. This isn't going well. And she's clearly not very interested, because she doesn't ask me anything. What if she decided I'm crap and walks off?

"And what do you do when you're not teaching or having drinks with strangers?" I ask jokingly. But she looks embarrassed. Shit, that was a really stupid thing to say.

"I… don't do this… very often", she says after another awkward silence. "In fact, it's the first time…"

"Really?" I'm about to tell her it's my first time too, when once again I remember James's advice. "Look confident and professional. Make it seem like you do it all the time, and you're good at it."

257

"I only moved to London a few weeks ago, and I don't know anyone here. Apart from the people at the school, but they don't know I'm…" She makes gestures as in you know what I mean, but I'm not actually sure if she means what I think she means, so I ask.

"A lesbian?" She gives me a horrified look, then looks down again and blushes. Is that an insult or something?

"Sorry, I just thought that's what you meant."

"That is what I meant. But I'm not… out. Yet. Where I come from, it's not a very common thing at all. It's quite… difficult."

"Oh, don't worry! This is London, everyone's accepted!" I say as though I were the town's ambassador. What the hell am I talking about anyway? God, I'm pissed.

"So, is it easy to be a lesbian here?"

"Sure. There are lots of places to hang out."

"Like, where?" Damn it, I should have done some research.

"Well… Soho's great. I usually go to mixed places, where men and straight people are allowed; although you don't see that many straight people in these places. Maybe it's because of the music."

"What's the music like?" What am I, the gay encyclopaedia?

"It's… varied", I say, trying to remember what on earth they play there. And then I have an idea. "Tell you what. Why don't I take you there?" Suddenly her face lights up.

"Really?"

"Yeah! Why not? It's only about half an hour on the train from here, isn't it?"

"We could get a cab, it'd be much quicker."

"I don't have enough for a cab."

"I'll pay!" she says, clearly excited. So we finish our drinks and jump in a taxi. I take her to First Out, which is packed with women, and at first, she's hesitant at going in.

"I don't know... I'm not wearing the right things."

"Oh don't be silly! There's no dress code! Come on, let's get some drinks!" I take her to the bar, and she insists on buying me an expensive wine. The music is rather awful, a mix of dance and R&B, but she seems to enjoy it. It's quite nice to be a guide; I'm introducing her to a whole new world. As we go back to the bar for more drinks, I nearly have a heart attack: the woman who spoke to me in G.A.Y. is standing right next to me. She raises her eyebrows and walks off.

"What's wrong? Do you know her?"

"Y... Yeah." I'm not gay, I remember saying that night. Shit, what if she talks to Stephanie? "She's... an ex."

"Really?" She sounds surprised. Oh God, I hope I haven't blown my cover!

"Yeah. Nasty break-up. She hates me now. Goes round telling people strange things about me."

"Huh. It's funny, I didn't think she'd be your type."

"What do you think is my type?" Please don't say men!

"Someone a bit more feminine. And prettier." I sigh in relief.

"Really?"

"Yeah. Someone like her", she says pointing at a rather attractive tall girl with long blond hair.

"Wow. I'd never have thought she was gay."

"Why not? You're pretty much the same, except not blonde."

"Y… Yes, I suppose so. Excuse me, I have to use the loo." I run to the toilets, hoping that by the time I get back, she'll have forgotten about it. Thankfully, she doesn't seem interested in my taste in women anymore, and we enjoy a few light-hearted conversations. She turns out to be a really nice person, who's even more insecure than I am. I never thought that'd be possible! At about 2:00am, we decide to call it a night.

"I've got to get some money out", she says as we leave the bar. Then she hands me a bunch of bank notes. "I've worked out it comes to around £350." I stare at the money in shock. I was having so much fun and getting so drunk, I completely forgot I was getting paid for it. Three hundred and fifty pounds. That's a month's rent.

"Thanks… but I can't." She looks at me in disbelief.

"Why not?"

"Because… it's not fair."

"I don't understand."

"You can't pay me for going to the pub with you. It's just not right. I'd feel like I've used you."

"But that was the plan. We both knew the deal."

"Well, I've changed my mind."

"Are you sure?"

"Yeah", I say biting my lips. She smiles.

"You're very kind."

"I don't know about that. You just caught me on a good day."

****

"Tell me you're joking!" James says, looking aghast.

"I'm not."

"Well, you're obviously even crazier than I thought."

"I couldn't take advantage of her loneliness."

"Why not?"

"Because that's immoral!"

"Darling, when it comes to money, it's always immoral. You just lost three hundred and fifty pounds. Three hundred and fifty pounds!"

"I had a nice evening. She's really friendly."

"I don't care if she's Mother bloody Theresa! It's not the point. Ah well, that's the end of your escort career before it even started. Job Centre, here we come."

"It's not all… I've invited her to come out with us."

"What for?"

"Because she doesn't know anyone here."

"You should be a Samaritan, you know that? Did you tell her you don't do pussies?"

"You're so crude. No, I didn't tell her."

"Well that should be interesting. Are you going to pretend to like girls every time she's around?"

"No, I'll come clean next time I see her."

"I'm sure she'll be pleased to hear the good news. That's a good start to her new life in London, isn't it? Her one and only friend betraying her."

"Don't be such a drama queen. It's not a big deal."

"Have you not seen Fatal Attraction?"

"What are you talking about? That's got nothing to do with anything!"

"Hide your bunnies, that's all I say."

****

The Job Centre is possibly the scariest place I've ever been to. There are people everywhere, most of whom I wouldn't give the time of the day. Even the staff look like they've just got out of prison.

"Ms Stevenson?" An old Asian woman shouts. I follow her to her desk and take a seat. I sit silently whilst she reads my forms and occasionally looks up to ask questions I've already answered on paper, such as Why did you leave your job? and How much money are you looking for? So I say whatever I think will make her give me more money.

"Where will you be looking for work?"

"Err... Job Centre?" I say half jokingly. But to be honest, I don't really know.

"And where else?"

"I was hoping you'd tell me, actually."

"Newspapers? Internet? Agencies?"
"Yeah. That all sounds good." She gives me a strange look and writes something down on my form. "Can you... just tell me... what kind of newspaper I can find

jobs in? And on the internet?" She gives me another look and shakes her head.

"It depends what you want to do, doesn't it?"

"I don't really know…"

"How can I help you if you don't know what it is you want to do?" I shrug. "Can you type?"

"I can use a keyboard, if that's what you mean."

"Can you use Word? Excel? PowerPoint? What kind of experience do you have?"

"Not really. Word, a little bit. And I worked in Market Research, like it says on my form."

"Anything else?" I'm struggling not to explode.

"No."

"Come back in two weeks at the same time to sign in. And try to think about your career prospects." My career prospects. What career? I can't do anything. I can't even be a bloody escort. Maybe I should call Stephanie and ask her for my money. James worked out that with Housing and Council Tax benefits, I should be OK for a while. Plus he'll lend me some money if I'm really desperate. And if I'm on the verge of being homeless, I can always tell my parents. Although I'll avoid it for as long as I can. And anyway, I worked my arse off in that company; I deserve some time off. I should buy a book. To distract myself. I get the bus to Muswell Hill and walk around the shops, in search of something cheap to buy. As I can't find anything in the charity shops, in end up in the Muswell Hill Bookshop (whoever picked that name has clearly no imagination whatsoever). I browse through the Sales shelves, pick an old Maeve Binchy book reduced to a pound and head for the till. It takes me a while to realise who's behind the counter. It's Adam. He smiles, clearly as surprised as I am.

"What... what are you doing... here?"

"I work here."

"Oh. Yes, of course. You're behind the counter. How... how have you been?"

"Good, actually." And he looks it. He's put on a bit of weight, had his hair cut and is wearing clean and tidy clothes.

"What about you?"

"Yeah... good." He picks up my book. "It's... for my mother!"

"Nice choice."

"So... how long have you been working here?"

"About a month. After you left, I realised what a prick I was. I had to do something or I was going to lose it completely. So I pulled myself together."

"I can see that. It's... great. I'm really happy for you."

"What about you? How's your job?"

"It's... not my job anymore."

"I always thought you could do better. Not that what I'm doing here is particularly challenging, obviously."

"At least you work with books... You like books", I say dumbly.

"Yes, I suppose it could have been worse. You did me a favour, Melanie. Without you, I don't know where I would have ended." He looks into my eyes and smiles and it sends shivers down my spine. Now I remember why I loved him.

"Adam, are we going for lunch?" A girl who's just come in shouts.

"Yeah. Give me a minute." He puts my book in a bag, hands it to me and smiles again. "Without you, I wouldn't have met Zoë", he says, clearly referring to the girl at the door. Suddenly, I feel like crying.

"That's... great. Congratulations."

"It's still really early days. I can't quite believe it, to be honest. I still have my lows... But I try to remember how horrible I was to you and it really helps." Oh, I'm so glad to hear that. Bastard.

"That's... great", I repeat, shaking. "I'd better get going. Nice to see you again." I walk out of the shop, my eyes watering. It's not fair. Why does he get to move on and find someone else so quickly? And why couldn't he be like he is now when we were together? They're probably laughing at me now. Well, fuck him. Fuck his girlfriend, fuck Phil, fuck everyone!

****

Three days without antidepressants. I feel like my head's empty and I'm going to pass out every time I stand up. John said I shouldn't stop taking them so abruptly, but I don't care. What's the point in them? Like James said, they don't change who I am. And they don't make me happy anyway. It seems to be worse when I drink, but to be quite honest, I kind of like the feeling. I'm all floaty. I went out clubbing last night and felt so light I couldn't stop giggling. James thought I'd taken drugs! I pulled again. He wasn't even particularly attractive; but I needed the company. All I could think of was that I wanted to get back at Adam and hurt him. Which was a really stupid excuse to sleep with someone, because he'll never find out and even if he did, he probably wouldn't care. And the worst thing is, this guy, Ross, I think his name was (or was it Tony?), wouldn't go away until this morning, because he was "too tired". I had to pretend to go to work so he could leave. Sleeping with strangers is far easier than I thought; especially after two bottles of wine and double shots of vodka. And the ironic thing is, today's Valentine's Day. Adam is probably taking Zoë for a nice romantic dinner, with no thoughts whatsoever for me. We didn't even have a Valentine's Day. James is out on a "date" or something, so I'm sitting at home in front of Terminator, with a box of Quality Streets and a giant pack of Maltesers. I wonder if Naomi's spending the night with George, or if she's on her own too. I feel like calling her, but I don't want to seem too sad. Maybe if I hadn't ignored Michael, I'd have someone to hang out with tonight. When I think that all the time I was worrying about Adam, he was shagging someone else! He could have told me, that would have saved me a lot of grief. James was right. And now he has a job and I'm the one going on benefits! It's so ironic. After the film is finished, I go online, to the "Computer Hell" room, somehow hoping to find Simon there, or just anyone I've spoken to before. But their server is down, so I turn my PC back off and jump into bed with my bag of Maltesers. I wake up a few hours later with melted chocolate all over my face. At lunchtime, I get another tearful call from Naomi; George dumped her last night. I rush to her house, where I find her lying on the sofa with used tissues all over the floor.

"What happened?"

"We were supposed to have dinner. A nice, romantic meal, so that, for a couple of hours, we'd pretend things were going fine. He had to work, so he told me to meet him at the restaurant, La Mesange, remember it?"

"Err... yes", I say, blushing at the thought of my awful behaviour that day.

"Well, I waited and waited, like a twat. After half an hour, I called him and you know what? He was in the fucking pub, with his fucking mates! Apparently, he'd told me to meet him at eight, but I know he said seven because I put it in my diary."

"And even if he had said eight, what was he doing in the pub when he told you he'd be working?" I ask trying to be helpful and then realise it was probably not the best thing to say without rubbing it in her face.

"So I left the restaurant", she continues. "I was so embarrassed. When I came back he was lying on the sofa, completely pissed. So I chucked him out."

"Really? Where did he go?"

"His mate's, probably. He could be under a bridge, for all I care!"

"Well, you did the right thing. But you shouldn't put yourself through so much stress in your condition."

"Believe me, I wouldn't if I could help it!"

"How's it going, by the way?" I ask pointing at her belly.

"Fine, I guess. It's been kicking lots. And I've been having lots of cramps today."

"It's probably because of last night."

"Do me a favour, will you? Pass me that bottle behind you." She points at an opened bottle of wine on the floor.

"Nam, I don't know much about pregnancy and stuff, but I don't think that would be wise."

"Since when do you care about babies?" She snaps.

"I don't, but…"

"Give me it, then!" I'm quite shocked. She's supposed to be the sensible one, after all.

"How much have you been drinking since you got pregnant?" She sighs.

"Almost nothing. The last thing I need right now is you giving me a hard time!"

"I just don't want you to fuck up, or you'll be sorry later, when your baby has three arms."

"I really don't think it works like that", she giggles. "Oh, forget it!"

An hour later, I get a text from James asking me to go clubbing with him. Once Naomi has cheered up and promised not to touch any alcohol, I run back home, have a shower and meet him and a couple of his friends in a really expensive bar on Old Compton Street. It's packed, loud and people keep bumping into me. Plus, I'm pretty sure I'm the only girl there and some of the men give me odd looks, probably meaning "You don't belong here". I haven't received any money from the benefits office yet, so James has to pay for most of my drinks. I try to catch a few guys' eyes, but no one's remotely interested. Silly me, what do I expect in a gay bar? I feel really shitty. Even James seems off, for some reason. Thankfully, I eventually manage to drag him out of the bar and onto the club, but as we're about to get in, I got a call from Naomi. She's quite cheeky, I did tell her I was going out! I'm really not in the mood to listen to her whining again. I leave it ring and a few seconds later, she calls again.

"Helloooo?" I say dryly.

"Melanie?" Who else would it be? Joan of Arc?

"Yeeees."

"It's me... I'm... I'm...." Oh for God's sake.

"I'm sorry Nam, but I can't talk right now. I'll give you a call tomorrow. Whatever he's done now, remember he's just an arsehole and you're better off..."

"Please don't hang up! It's not about George... I... I... I think I'm giving birth. My waters broke."

"What are you talking about? You're not due for another month." She's so melodramatic sometimes. I bet she's just pissed herself without noticing.

"Well I think it's happening now, Mel! I'm so scared!" Now that I think of it, she did mention cramps earlier on. Oh God. Oh God!

"OK, keep calm. When did it start?"

"I don't know, an hour ago, maybe two?"

"What? Have you rung an ambulance?"

"Excuse me, are you going in or what?" Some guy behind me interrupts.

"Oh, sod off! No, not you Nam. Have you rung an ambulance?"

"No, not yet!"

"What the hell are you waiting for? Are you planning to give birth on your bloody carpet?"

"I'll... I'll do it now! Please, can you come with me?" James is standing by the door and making big "come on in" gestures at me. Damn it!

"I won't make it before the ambulance. What about your parents? Or George?"

"I can't get hold of them. And there's no way I'm asking him!"

"OK, OK. Ring an ambulance and I'll try to get to you as soon as I can. Please, don't panic. It's all going to be fine."

I make my way out of the queue and run in search of a cab, soon realising that I don't have any money whatsoever. So I walk back to the club, but James must have already gone in. I call an ambulance, just in case Naomi passed out or simply forgot and jump on the tube. But I get to her flat too late; there's no answer. I ask an old woman the address of the nearest hospital and try to figure out a way to get there, hoping that Naomi isn't just lying dead in her house. The thing is, I haven't got a bloody clue where that damn hospital is. I walk around pointlessly for about ten minutes, then decide to ask a bus driver. Turns out, I have to catch two different buses, and that is if I'm actually going to the right place. I arrive at the Greenwich Hospital over two hours after Naomi called me. Thankfully, this is the right hospital… but by the time I make it to her room, it's already over. I find her sitting on her bed, looking very tired but smiling.

"That was bloody quick! Aren't these things supposed to take a whole day?"

"Apparently it was one of the quickest deliveries they've had in a long time." I look around, realising there's no sign of the actual baby.

"Where is…"

"They took her for some tests. Just to make sure everything was OK, because she was early and everything." I can't help smiling.

"It's a girl?"

"Yes. I called her Thea."

"Thea? That's my…"

"Your middle name. I know. You can see her if you want." A nurse takes me to a room where half a dozen babies are lying in little incubators, with tubes in their nose.

"There she is. A beautiful, healthy baby, by the looks of things. She just couldn't wait to come out and see the world." As I look at Thea, her tiny body and pink skin, my eyes water. I stay there for ten, twenty minutes maybe, watching her sleep and occasionally move her little fingers and nostrils. I can't believe this minuscule vulnerable thing will grow up to be a person. I can't believe twenty-two years ago, this was me. And then, for the very first time in my life, I get that feeling I never thought capable of having. Maybe I can do this. Maybe my body, my head, are not all wrong. Maybe I don't need alcohol, short skirts and one-night stands. Maybe there's hope.

www.ingramcontent.com/pod-product-compliance
Lightning Source LLC
Chambersburg PA
CBHW031150270326
41931CB00006B/214